HOW TO HAVE

Great
sex

FOR THE REST OF YOUR LIFE

About the Authors

Val Sampson and Julia Cole are experienced journalists who have both worked with couples and written books on sexual issues. Val Sampson has written for many leading newspapers and magazines. Her latest book was the best-selling *Tantra: The Art of Mind-Blowing Sex*. Julia Cole is a leading psychosexual therapist; her latest book was *How to Stay Together Forever*.

HOW TO HAVE

Great
sex

FOR THE REST OF YOUR LIFE

VAL SAMPSON
& JULIA COLE

PIATKUS

Copyright © 2004 by Val Sampson and Julia Cole

First published in Great Britain in 2004 by
Piatkus Books Ltd
5 Windmill Street
London W1T 2JA
e-mail: info@piatkus.co.uk

The moral right of the authors has been asserted

A catalogue record for this book is available from the British Library

ISBN 0 7499 2547 7

This book has been printed on paper manufactured with respect for the environment using wood from managed sustainable resources

Edited by Jan Cutler
Text design by Paul Saunders

Typeset by Palimpsest Book Production Limited, Polmont, Stirlingshire
Printed and bound in Great Britain by Mackays of Chatham plc, Chatham, Kent

To my parents, Irene and John, for their love,
support and friendship
Val Sampson

For Tricia Cosford, my friend and mentor
Julia Cole

contents

introduction

Sex in long-term relationships is regarded by most of us as the equivalent of Cinderella before she meets her Prince: unglamorous, dutiful and definitely not exciting. Newspapers, TV and magazines focus mainly on dating and new relationships with a nod in the direction of recovering from bust-ups and divorce. Sex after 15 years of marriage is not big news. As far as most of the media is concerned, when the first flush of excitement and hormones dies down, you are on your own.

How to Have Great Sex for the Rest of Your Life will help you in the previously uncharted territory of sex once the novelty has worn off. There are hundreds of thousands of couples in Britain, if not millions of us, who have no wish to end our relationships, but who are nevertheless living with sex lives that are dwindling, disappointing or non-existent. Added to this is a feeling of isolation and being out of step with everyone else. In a society that is overloaded with overtly sexual images it is easy to imagine that the rest of the world is having great sex, and it's only you and your partner whose bedroom highlight is a cup of tea and a really good book.

So if sex in your marriage is less exciting than it could be, don't be disheartened. The message of this book is that you can change this simply, powerfully and enjoyably. Not only can you rekindle your sex life, if that is what you desire, but also the sex you can have with your partner in a long-term relationship can be transformed into the best sex of your life. No matter what your age or the number of years you have been together. All you need to do is to be open to looking at yourself, and at your partner, and to be willing to make some changes. It might be useful if you begin to think now about how you would like your sex life to be as you start to read this book. What will you be doing when you have the sex life you really want? How will you be treating your partner and how will they be responding to you?

Perhaps the first point to make is that sex doesn't necessarily matter to everyone. There are couples leading non-sexual lives together that are creative, fulfilling and very happy. Companionship and kindness is all they seek from each other and they have every right to expect respect from other people for the choice they have made.

But for many, celibacy is an enforced option, inflicted on one partner by another who has gone off sex and is probably hoping the whole problem will simply disappear if he or she ignores it for long enough. If this is your situation, there is hope and a way to resolve the situation without bitterness or recriminations.

One of the biggest illusions in our society's attitude to sex is that we think of it as though it is somehow 'outside' the rest of our relationship. Indeed, we often think of sex as though it is 'outside' ourselves, and as such almost becomes yet another problem we have to solve. In fact, sex is simply our response to another person and the world around us. We don't need to worry about 'failing' at sex and not managing to meet the media's complicated requirements. Real sex is about fine-tuning ourselves, and becoming more in touch with our physical and emotional responses to other people, and our partner in particular.

So this book is not solely about different sex positions or breathing techniques to ensure a bigger and better orgasm (although you will find some helpful tips you might like to try). Actually having great sex for the rest of your life means accepting that your sex life and your relationship with your partner are inextricably bound together. After all, the act of sex inevitably involves a relationship between two people (even if that relationship is only a one-night stand). You will need to think about the way you interact with each other outside the bedroom if anything is to change inside it.

The following eight chapters examine relationship issues like trust, self-esteem and one of the biggest hurdles to a flourishing sex life: parenting. Not all of these may apply to you – feel free to dip in and out of the chapters according to your inclination. You will find that each chapter is written by two authors: the first half is a general introduction to the subject by Val Sampson, and the second half, by Julia Cole, offers a practical guide to steps you can take to make changes in your own sex life, along with useful stories illustrating the impact of these changes on the lives of other people.

We are both authors who have worked with couples and have written books about sexual issues. We share a vision of sex that is exciting, passionate and committed, which brings us to the issue of why we think sex matters in a relationship.

3

We believe a rewarding sex life is important for a couple at all stages of their lives because sex is the one thing you do together that marks out your relationship as different and special. In our busy existence we find ourselves giving time to our work, our children and our friends. All too often our partners end up at the bottom of a long to-do list – sometimes below walking the dog and emptying out the dustbin.

Taking time to make love with a partner automatically places them back at the top of your list, which is where they rightly belong. If you cast your mind back to when you first met and fell in love, remember the priority they took, sometimes over your friends, and invariably above the household chores. But several years (or even months) down the line, and it is easy to treat them like a well-worn sofa, as a comfortable part of the furniture. Having great sex with them is a reminder to you both of the valuable and unique role you play as lovers in each other's lives.

Sex does not always have to be 'amazing', 'sensational' or even extremely passionate. And if your sex life isn't described by those adjectives, there is nothing wrong with you. It is fine to have sex that is funny, cosy and comforting. If, on the other hand, you feel your sex life is none of the above and that 'dull and unfulfilling', or even 'non-existent', is the most accurate summary, then this book will help you gain a new perspective on the choices you can make in your relationship that will change things for the better.

If you are hoping to rekindle a sex life that has petered out over the years, don't necessarily expect to have great sex the moment you begin again. You may have to work your way through nervous and tentative sex before you reach a place where some of the suggestions in this book feel like they might become natural to you. This is perfectly normal. Great sex is a combination of skills, patience, love and enthusiasm. Don't expect to go from zero to ten out of ten if you are out of practice. To begin, focus on what does work for you and concentrate on that.

We believe that men and women can experience sex differently, and that although women have made huge strides in gaining equality in the workplace, a sexual relationship is not suited to a strict division of labour along the lines of 'anything you can do, I can do better'.

Increasing numbers of women are adopting the 'love 'em and leave 'em' approach to casual sex that used to be more usually the preserve of men. Whereas this may suit some individuals, most people eventually seek a fulfilling, long-term relationship with a partner that will meet their emotional needs as well as their physical ones. This book is written with them in mind.

Generally, men and women have different sexual responses. It is as if a man comes to the boil like a kettle, while a woman simmers like a pan of water. Of course, this is a generalisation, and no two people share exactly the same sexual characteristics. Similarly, our sexual response can alter with the length of time that we have known our partner. But for too long our usual modern pattern of sex has emulated the male model of the sprint towards orgasm, and some women have either been made to feel guilty or that there is something lacking in them if they don't achieve orgasm as quickly and efficiently as the majority of men.

On a practical level, in some of the chapters we suggest using lubricant and possibly a vibrator in your sexual relationship. This is for the simple reason that many couples give up on sex, either because it becomes physically uncomfortable or because the woman finds it difficult to reach a climax.

(Nature has made it much easier for a man to have an orgasm than a woman.) If there are no underlying physical or emotional reasons limiting your sexual pleasure, the addition of a little lubricant can make sex much more enjoyable for both of you. And the introduction of a vibrator, which practically guarantees an orgasm for a woman, can take the pressure off both of you from time to time.

Use a water-based lubricant rather than an oil-based one; you can pick up a tube of KY jelly, for example, with your supermarket shopping. These days you can buy a vibrator on the high street, although we recommend the range designed by Julia available from www.emotionalbliss.com.

Focusing on the female sexual response and a more female-friendly approach to sex is something that the best male lovers do naturally. They deserve huge amounts of praise for this, as they have practically no role models to draw on. Pornographic books and films (which are the source of most men's sex education) are aimed to encourage male masturbation rather than a genuine understanding of human sexuality. Even the thrusting in porn movies is deliberately timed to the masturbatory rhythm of a male hand. It bears very little relation to what most women appreciate in real life.

For this reason, *How to Have Great Sex for the Rest of Your Life* is going to fly the flag for a different kind of sexual interaction between men and women. But is certainly not about female pleasure at the expense of male satisfaction. Both men and women who make time for sex that involves intimacy and connection as well as physical pleasure discover a way of being together that can't be bettered. And we don't insist that you give up doing what you already find enjoyable and fun – whatever that might be. This book is about opening a door on another way of thinking about sex that you may not have encountered before.

After all, if Cinderella and her Prince did live happily ever after, they needed to learn how to make love with each other after they had children and taken on responsibility for the ageing King. And when the romance of the ball and glass slipper was just a distant memory.

desire and libido

. . . .

Sexual desire is one of the most powerful of all human experiences. The potent combination of mental and physical chemistry has the ability to transform the way we feel about ourselves, and our partners. Many people compare it to the high of an illicit drug. It is a heightened state of excitement and physical awareness. Simply to brush against the hand of the person you desire can send shock waves through your body.

Feeling no desire at all

So there are few things more disheartening in a relationship than feeling no desire for your partner at all. And, sadly, climbing into bed with someone whose touch leaves you cold, or, even worse, whose sexual advances make your heart sink, is a depressingly common occurrence for couples in long-term relationships.

Why sex surveys can be unhelpful

Lots of people who are worried about their loss of desire anxiously seek statistics about how often 'the average' couple makes love. The results of these surveys of couples' sex lives vary hugely according to the circumstances of the research and the honesty of the individuals answering the questions. Broadly speaking, they are unhelpful. Beating yourself up because Mr and Mrs Average have sex three times a week and you are lucky to manage once a month probably isn't the information you need if you want to change things for the better in your own love life. (And, of course, who's to say that Mr and Mrs Average don't have dull, unrewarding three-minute sex three times a week, whereas the couple that make love once every month take their time to really enjoy it, ensure each other's pleasure, and find their occasional sex life entirely satisfying?)

There's no RDA for sex

The government have not issued a recommended daily allowance (RDA) for sex, so perhaps a useful first step is to liberate yourself from the idea that in some way you are failing to measure up. Similarly, if you are feeling rather smug about the sheer number of times you have sex with your partner, don't pat yourself on the back until you can honestly say that usually the quality of the experience matches the high quantity of the times you make love.

Desire and libido

Before we continue to talk about desire, it's useful to explain the difference between desire and libido – terms that are often mixed up and used interchangeably.

What is desire?

Desire is a psychological state, influenced by a range of factors, including your upbringing, and the culture you grew up in. If you were a woman in certain parts of Africa, for example, you may be conditioned by your culture to fancy a bloke with an elaborately painted face. In traditional Australian Aboriginal culture, younger men revered older women, and the average Edwardian male lusted after a woman with a big bust and even bigger bustle that drew attention to her bottom. Doubtless, for an Edwardian woman, a man responding 'yes' to her question 'Does my bum look big in this?' was a great compliment.

Often people have mixed feelings about experiencing sexual desire, especially if they grew up in a family where any discussion of sex was frowned on, or sex was regarded as something dirty and unpleasant. But this need not be a barrier to embracing the gift of sexuality and letting it shine. (Later in this chapter, Julia offers some ideas for reframing past experiences that will help to get you back on track and more able to enjoy the pleasure that feeling sexual desire can bring.)

So what is libido?

The term 'libido' should refer to a person's sex drive. It is more of a combination of brain chemicals and physiology. Some people are born with a high libido, others have a libido they barely notice, and although external factors can influence both extremes, your libido is partly a question of genetics and the make-up of your own body.

Hormones play a critical role in your libido. Women and men produce testosterone – the hormone that regulates your sex drive. Some women tend to produce more of it around the time of ovulation, and that is when they feel at their most sexy, others seem more interested in sex during the first half of their menstrual cycle when their oestrogen levels are increased, boosting a sense of well-being.

In the past it was thought that it was only women whose attitudes and behaviour were affected by their hormones. Now we know than men can be slaves to their hormones too. A man's testosterone level can double in the morning, for example. And a study of men submerged in a nuclear submarine for months at a time saw them experience periods of increased beard growth, accompanied by noticeable mood swings from euphoria to mild depression. Researchers attributed these changes to a previously unobserved four- to six-week testosterone cycle.

Having said this, however, a dip in a man's testosterone level is probably not enough to reduce his interest in sex. Most men have more than enough testosterone to sustain their interest in sex, even when they are on the low end of a cycle. For women, though, it is a different picture.

Research suggests that the testosterone level of many women dips below a critical threshold at regular intervals throughout the month, diminishing or even eliminating their interest in sex. Some women have such low levels that they never desire sex, even when their hormones are at peak levels.

The point to remember here, though, is that sex is not just about biology. Even if you are a woman with a low libido, perhaps as a result of having a low level of testosterone, it does not necessarily follow that you will never be interested in sex. You may meet a man who treats you in such a way that you are frequently filled with desire for him and your sex life is blissful. Hormones are simply part of the complex jigsaw that makes up our sexual response.

So both libido and desire play important roles in your sexuality. A quote from Woody Allen's classic movie *Annie Hall*, starring Diane Keaton, offers a humorous example of a couple with a mismatched level of desire and differing libidos. Woody and Diane are seen being asked by their psychotherapists how often they have sex:

WOODY 'Hardly ever. Maybe three times a week.'
DIANE 'Constantly. I'd say three times a week.'

As you can see, sex becomes a problem only when either of you, or both of you, see it as such. If one or other of you isn't happy, then it is time to take stock and address the issue. If, on the other hand, you have an infrequent sex life, but both of you are happy with it, and with all the other aspects of your lives together, then you have nothing to worry about.

Losing interest

It is important to remember that it is perfectly normal to lose interest in sex for several weeks at a time. Sexual desire ebbs and flows in all of us, it is not a constant. Certainly as we grow older, we can experience shifts in our patterns of desire. Men may find the need to make love is less urgent, whereas women find liberation from worrying about unwanted pregnancy after the menopause allows their interest in sex to flourish.

A failing libido

There are physical reasons for a failing libido, anything from eczema to thyroid disorders and diabetes can affect your sex drive, and individuals who suffer from depression can find that their libido disappears altogether. Rather unfairly, anti-depressants also quash sexual feelings, as do antibiotics, drugs for heart disease and high blood pressure, as well as an array of over-the-counter drugs including antihistamines and even some cold and flu remedies.

If you suddenly experience a loss of libido, and there are no other problems in your relationship, it is worth getting your GP's opinion before your sex life goes into decline. Quite apart from the fact that there may be an underlying health problem that needs attention, acting fast to get help prevents the 'no-sex rot' setting in. This is when couples stop having sex for a specific reason, whether it is to do with health or a family crisis, and then when that problem is resolved, their sex life doesn't get back into gear.

Look up to seven years younger

'Use it or lose it' applies to your sexuality as much as your levels of fitness. A barren patch in a couple's sex life can become a desert surprisingly quickly once you begin to neglect each other physically. If you are looking for encouragement to keep your sex life going, listen to Dr David Weeks, the head of Old Age Psychology at the Royal Edinburgh Hospital and author of *Superyoung – the proven way to stay young forever*. He says that people who look, act and often feel far younger than their chronological age tend to have sex more often. Improving the quality of your sex life, he says, can help make you look up to seven years younger. An orgasm not only releases beta endorphins – natural painkillers which alleviate anxiety – it also triggers the release of human growth hormone, which plays a role in reducing fatty tissues and increasing lean muscle in various parts of the body, leading to a more youthful appearance.

Sex is good for you

Certainly, sex is a healthier option than cosmetic surgery when it comes to staying youthful. (It also boosts your immune system by as much as 20 per cent.) But what if you can understand the benefits of having sex on an intellectual level, but your desire to have sex has disappeared?

How to rekindle desire

Without desire, sex becomes a chore, like shopping or cleaning. It is just something else that needs to be ticked off the list of jobs to be done. If you have been having regular desire-free sex for a while, expect to go off sex altogether fairly soon. Sex does not always have to be about wild passion, but to be satisfactory it does have to be an experience that both parties enjoy on some level. Otherwise, why do it?

There are, of course, many answers to this. People have sex out of anger, fear, jealousy, and even out of sympathy for their partner. But if you are looking to relocate your sense of desire for your partner, you need to stand back from your relationship for a moment, and ask yourself: *are you prepared to make a decision to desire your partner?*

Making a decision to desire

Once the initial infatuation with each other wears off, which it inevitably will (usually within 18 months of being together), you can no longer rely on the initial rush of love chemicals, which nature arranges to bond you to each other at first.

We might be programmed to have sex in order to reproduce, but we are not programmed to have exciting, stimulating, emotionally intimate sex – these things we have to work at and to create with each other. For a couple in a long-term relationship, the pattern of sexual closeness is the reversal of the way things were when they initially got together.

Sexual attraction to someone new is usually instant and powerful. Lust takes over, you have sex, which is often fast and exciting, and you may want to talk later. Very little mental effort is involved, nearly everything happens on the physical level. Once you have been together for a while, though, this pattern shifts. And it is here that a lot of people get stuck. When the novelty and excitement of sex with someone they have fallen in love with starts to fade, either they worry that perhaps they didn't really love their partner in the first place, or they sadly shrug their shoulders and think 'that's the way it goes'.

Fortunately, there is an even more fulfilling path ahead, but it requires a degree of effort and determination to find it. Firstly, you have to invest some time in your relationship. You can no longer rely on being spontaneous. Those who wait to be inspired before they have sex, have very little sex. But just because you plan to have sex with your partner, it does not mean that the experience has to be second-rate. There are very few things in life that aren't improved, in fact, with a little planning, and sex is no exception to this. And, of course, deciding to plan when to make love does not mean that you can no longer be spontaneous as well.

When you were first dating

Think back to when you were first dating. Then you spent hours getting ready to meet, you wondered what you might talk about together, and you made an effort to make them smile. You may not have been consciously planning to have sex with your date, but unconsciously you were investing heavily in the time you spent together. Now you need to put in a similar amount of effort. However, to achieve equally good results, it needs to be focused in a slightly different way.

For sex to be more than a routine, you need to connect with your partner on an emotional and mental level. This means being prepared to be intimate with them. For the purpose of rekindling desire, it means being open about your emotions and feelings and not being afraid that you will be rejected because of this. Women tend to find this easier than men, who are often reluctant to appear vulnerable emotionally. But you don't have to go overboard and spill all your deepest fears in order to have good sex long term.

Communication-starved women/ sex-starved men

You do genuinely have to listen to what your partner is saying, though, and be willing to share what's going on in your head, too. For some reason, women often want sex after they have done this and are feeling emotionally close and supported by their partner. Men, on the other hand, tend to feel more connected to their partner after sex. The worst of all worlds in long-term relationships is the all-too-common scenario of communication-starved women and sex-starved men.

Understanding differences

It is important to bear in mind these different male and female responses when you make the decision to rekindle your desire for your partner. Understanding differences goes a long way to accepting and working with them. So if you are looking to fan the embers of your sex life into a blaze, you can begin by planning a time and place when you can have sex, and talk to your partner at a deeper, more emotional level than normal beforehand. Again, this doesn't have to be about raising your deepest, darkest secrets. Just give them a clue about your emotional reaction to some of the things that are going on in your lives. If you aren't sure what your emotional reactions are, be honest, and say. Just be prepared to give a little of yourself to your partner.

Don't expect miracles when you first make a date to make love. In fact, it is far better if you keep your expectations low and focus on the little things that do work, rather than what you feel doesn't work. Trust that things will start to improve, and you are on the right track.

Keep touching

In the meantime, keep touching each other. This sounds ridiculously simply advice, but it is remarkable how many couples no longer touch each other when they stop having sex. For some, any touch in this situation becomes loaded with sexual significance and this can make either party feel uncomfortable or resentful. But touch is one of our most basic needs. Babies deprived of touch fail to thrive; adults don't fare much better.

Scientists have proved that women who are denied regular, affectionate touch become depressed and less interested in sex, whereas men who miss out on tender touching become more aggressive and uninterested in touch that is not sexual. When we touch each other, a hormone called oxytocin is released into the bloodstream, decreasing stress levels and increasing sex hormones. In women this raises sexual responsiveness and in men it boosts the sensitivity of their penis and improves their erection.

Simply holding hands to begin with when you are sitting and watching TV, or walking side by side, is a good way to begin to touch each other. Kissing each other hello and goodbye is also something that can simply be forgotten, especially if you have young children and are physically involved in caring for them. It is easy for them to absorb your 'affection' energy. However, we don't have limited amounts of affection to dispense, and remembering to regularly kiss our partners in a sexual way is a reminder of the unique role they play as our lovers.

Awakening physical desire on your own

Sometimes you have to wake up your body gently, sexually speaking. It is hard to rekindle a sexual relationship with your partner if as an individual you aren't in touch with your sexuality at all. Begin to masturbate two or three times a week. This isn't a problem for most men as their sexual equipment is close to hand, but some women find it difficult if they have never done it before.

Always use a water-based lubricant, as this will enhance the sensation and should make it a much more pleasurable experience. Find somewhere warm and comfortable where you won't be disturbed, think about a person or an incident you find arousing and begin to stroke the whole of your body. Gradually focus on your clitoris, rubbing it slowly and tenderly in small circles, and keeping a steady rhythm. Some women find that touching their nipples at the same time is even more arousing. It may take anything between five and 15 minutes to reach orgasm; some women take longer. If you want quicker results, invest in a vibrator.

A tip for 'female friendly' penetration

When you do begin to make love with your partner again, it is helpful if a man remembers that it is the first three inches of his partner's vagina that experiences the most sensation.

The Kama Sutra may include some positions that might make you more amused than amorous, but it does have some excellent advice when it comes to the way a man penetrates a woman. If you are man, instead of simply pumping in and out (sexual behaviour that leaves a lot of women examining cracks in the ceiling or wondering if it's time to change the bed sheets), circle your hips in what is literally a 'screwing' motion. This is much more enjoyable for your partner as it is far more likely to reach her most sensitive places. And if you are looking for an even more enthusiastic reaction, try the grandly named 'Thrusts of the Phoenix'. This is where you enter her shallowly for eight thrusts and go in deep on the ninth. Most women love this, and for some it is the best way to reach an orgasm during intercourse.

Also bear in mind that most women need at least 20 minutes of foreplay to be fully aroused before they are ready for sex. One of the joys of growing older is that a man's urgent need to ejaculate diminishes. This often leads to the exciting discovery that there is as much fun to be had for both of you en route to orgasm as there is in reaching the final destination.

For women

A woman's PC muscle connects the front of the pelvis to the lower spine. It is the muscle you rely on when you are desperate to go to the loo, but have to hold on. If you have had a baby, it is the muscle you feel most acutely when you push out in childbirth. The PC muscle is one of the main movers and shakers during orgasm, and if you learn to use it properly, you strengthen your ability not only to give your partner a more enjoyable time when he is inside you but also to expand orgasmic sensations too.

Like all muscles, the PC benefits from exercise. Firstly, try tightening and relaxing it in short bursts. Tighten it as you inhale, then relax it as you breathe out. Do this 20 times a day.

When you feel comfortable with this, progress to tightening with the in-breath, retaining the breath for six seconds, and then bearing down as you exhale. If this feels too much like hard work, stick to the tightening and relaxing. As long as you do it every day you should notice a difference in your love-making within a couple of months. (It also means that you are far less likely to suffer from incontinence as you grow older.)

For men

Like women, men have a group of muscles from the pubic bone (pubo) in the front of their body to the tailbone or coccyx (coccygeus) in the back. Some cultures believe that a man who uses his PC muscle properly can contract it when he is on the threshold of an orgasm and delay ejaculation. If practised sufficiently, he can go on to experience an orgasm without ejaculating at all.

Broadly speaking, men can exercise their PC muscle in the same way as women. Men, however, are most aware of it when they are trying to push out the last few drops of urine. If you have a strong PC muscle, you should be able to stop the flow of urine midstream and then start it again. If you have trouble doing this, the chances are your PC muscle is weak and could do with some exercise. Stopping the flow of urine may sting at first. This is normal, and should stop within a couple of weeks. If it doesn't, you might have an infection and should visit your GP to sort it out.

Exercise your PC muscle by stopping and starting urinating, between three and six times, or as many times as you can manage. Or if you feel this will earn you strange looks in the Gents, simply inhale and tense your PC muscle and exhale and release it ten times, and repeat at least two or three times a day. The joy of this is that it is an exercise you can do anywhere – in your car, on the train or picking up your email. Don't push yourself too hard, though. The PC muscle is like any other in that if you over-exercise, it will become sore and uncomfortable.

Viagra

Any discussion of desire and libido in the 21st century needs to include Viagra, the drug that enables men who could not achieve reliable erections to have firm erections once more. The launch of Viagra in 1998 has changed the lives of millions, and it is the fastest-selling drug in history.

Nine little blue pills are dispensed worldwide every second, and sales are estimated at US$1.5 billion. Whereas Viagra was originally marketed to help men suffering from erectile dysfunction, there have been stories in newspapers and magazines about healthy men and even some women who have been taking it to pep up their sex lives. Medical advice is that you should not take Viagra without a prescription, and if lack of desire is your problem, taking Viagra is not a solution.

Viagra works by increasing blood flow to the sexual organs, and while this may increase the sexual confidence of a man who had previously doubted his ability to gain an erection, Viagra does not come with a set of instructions on how to handle the impact it will have on your relationship. For every couple that has delightedly resumed making love thanks to Viagra, there is probably at least one other where resuming a previously abandoned sex life has been fraught with emotional difficulties.

Very little research has so far been done into the impact of Viagra on partnerships, but it seems unlikely that a pill alone will magically restore anyone's sex life without the need for some extra communication between the couple concerned.

Viagra also re-emphasises the role of penetrative sex, which has an important role in love-making, but *sex is not just about penetration* (or a sprint towards orgasm).

Already the drug industry is trying to find an equally lucrative drug for the newly discovered syndrome of Female Sexual Dysfunction. While anyone paying serious attention to women's sexual problems is to be applauded, researchers looking for the female equivalent of Viagra have hit a stumbling block. The fact is women's sexuality is complex; one of the most critical issues being how a woman feels about her relationship.

A man with an erection is usually ready to have sex; more factors come into play for a woman if she is to be filled with desire for her partner. Someone once said that communication is the best lubrication for many women, and it is hard to imagine scientists managing to provide that in pill form.

Rediscover your sexual drive and desire

As you will have read in the first half of this chapter, sex drive and desire can be affected by many different issues: your hormonal balance, illness, stress and relationship problems, to mention just a few. But you can keep your sexual desire alive through a willingness to explore new ways of thinking about intimacy and by committing to work on your personal sexuality.

The following case study about Mike and Liz explores the most common causes and responses to loss of desire. It's likely you will recognise some of their concerns if you also feel you have 'gone off sex'. After Mike and Liz's story, look at the ideas and suggestions for boosting your own sexual desire. They are designed to help you feel more in touch with your sexual needs and desires.

CASE STUDY ·

Mike and Liz

Mike and Liz have been together five years. They have lived together for three years and married two years ago. Six months before they married, Mike had a 'one-night stand' with an old girl-friend. When she discovered, three weeks later, Liz's initial feeling was that they might break up. Mike felt terrible about the fling, which had been mainly fuelled by too much booze on a lads' night out, and apologised to Liz, telling her it would never happen again. Liz forgave him and they stayed together. But Liz felt differently about their sex life from then on, tracing the start of her loss of interest in sex back to this time. Their wedding, six months after the affair, boosted their sex life for a time, but the frequency of their love-making has declined a great deal – from twice a week at the start of their relationship to about once every six weeks – and Liz feels that she is not fully present when they make love. She describes this feeling as an 'out of body experience'. 'I'm having sex, but not really involved. It's as if I'm not really there.'

Mike has taken promotion at work since he and Liz got married and works longer hours now that he is in a managerial position. He often feels very tired and flops on the sofa at the end of the day with a can of lager and the sport on TV. He would like to make love more often but is finding it difficult to summon up the energy to spend much time thinking about it. He and Liz now have sex that is a ten-minute fumble at the end of the day rather than the hour-long love-making sessions they enjoyed at the start of their partnership. He still feels guilty about his fling, and knows that Liz was badly affected by it, but he also knows he loves her and doesn't want anyone else. He has found it hard to say this to Liz, as he is wary of raising the subject again, telling himself it is better to 'let things lie'.

As a result, Liz and Mike have found they don't feel particularly sexy or interested in sex with each other. Liz wonders if Mike has gone off her, while Mike tries to forget the whole issue. They have begun to avoid situations where sex might be on the agenda, such as opportunities for early nights or at quiet weekends. Mike often stays up watching TV until he thinks Liz is asleep, whereas Liz has stopped being affectionate towards Mike. Both of them feel switched off sex and not sure how to rekindle the feelings they once had towards each other. They rationalise this by thinking 'it's what happens when you are in a long-term relationship'. Liz has friends with the same problems and they have even joked together about preferring a bar of chocolate to sex. Nevertheless, secretly both of them would like to be closer and for sex to have the passion it once had.

* *

Liz and Mike's story contains many of the elements that cause trouble with libido and desire. They suffered a relationship crisis that has not been fully discussed; they are frequently tired and have begun to avoid sex. These problems are causing a vicious circle: anxiety about sex, leading to lack of sex that makes them more anxious. So what can you do to break this cycle and improve sexual desire? The rest of this chapter suggests ways to tackle low desire and improve sexual responsiveness.

First things first

It is not possible to feel sexy if you are coping with hidden concerns about your relationship. Many couples think they can somehow excise their sex life from other events in their relationship or life. But how you feel about sex is linked to your general day-to-day life. Here are some questions to ask yourself about your relationship and yourself.

Am I angry?

Anger can cause you to switch off your sexual desire. You may not necessarily be angry with your partner, but angry about a situation at work, with a relative or friend. Anger that bubbles away inside you (as in Liz's anger at Mike's affair) can stop you wanting sex because it prevents you relaxing and feeling able to trust. If you are angry with your partner, you are likely to avoid lovemaking because you may not want to appear emotionally vulnerable with someone who could take advantage of this openness. Chronic anger can depress feelings of desire for years, meaning that sex is off-limits most of the time.

Coping with anger

● *Trace the origin of your anger.* Ask yourself why you feel this way. For example, if you feel annoyed that your partner has not noticed how difficult you are finding it to care for children and work full time, you need to talk to them about what you need. The hope that a partner will also be an expert mind-reader can often account for misunderstandings and feelings of frustration that lead to unexpressed anger.

● *Be practical and specific about what you feel.* Avoid woolly statements about 'feeling annoyed'. Say what you feel angry about and explain why this issue has caused you to feel aggrieved.

● *Look for practical solutions.* For example, if you feel your partner is not affectionate towards you, ask for a kiss and cuddle when you get into bed together or a kiss goodbye as he or she goes off to work.

There is more in-depth help on anger and sexual feelings in Chapter 6, Anger.

Am I anxious?

Worrying about anything can stop you feeling sexy. This is because anxiety produces feelings of lack of safety and reduces concentration – both key elements for a good sex life. If you are worrying about work or money, children or a sick relative, for example, your natural interest in sex will diminish. Forcing yourself to have sex when you feel this way can be detrimental and ruin the sense of closeness so important to love-making. It is better to try to sort out your anxiety than suppress it.

Coping with anxiety

● **Work out what you are worrying about.** This may sound obvious advice. If you are worrying, of course you know what it is. But you may be worrying on a wider scale about a number of issues. Take a notepad and pen and write down what you think you are concerned about. For example, if your general worry is money, write this as a heading. Now list everything you are concerned about. Pick the one item that you feel lies at the root of the list.

● **Take practical steps to resolve it.** For example, if you worry about unexpected bills coming in, work out whether you could put cash aside to cope with this issue. Talk to your partner about your worries. A worry shared really is a worry halved.

● **Give yourself a worry limit.** If you find yourself worrying about vague or unspecific issues, such as falling ill or your children's future, allow yourself to worry for a specified time each day. An hour is probably enough. Decide you will think about your concerns between 6.00 and 7.00 p.m. only. If you find yourself worrying at other times, tell yourself 'I'll save that for my worry hour'. Interestingly this method can diminish worrying as you may find you forget to worry at the time you have set aside!

Am I tired?

Tiredness is probably the number-one desire killer. If you feel exhausted, fulfilling sex will be the last thing on your mind. Instead, you may only crave sleep or rest. If you feel that your tiredness is partly caused by your partner, perhaps because they do not help with household chores, childcare, or because you work long hours to support your family, you may have a mixture of tiredness and discontent to cope with.

Coping with tiredness

● *Assess your lifestyle*. Are you charging about trying to be superwoman or superman? It is crucial to find at least an hour a day when you can relax and let go for a while. If you slump in front of the TV every evening, put aside some time to listen to relaxing music, take a long, warm bath or a peaceful cup of tea. Avoid drinking excessive amounts of alcohol or taking drugs to help you relax as these can often have long-term side effects. (If you are a woman drinking more than two glasses of wine each night – or a man drinking over three glasses – you are over the safe weekly alcohol limit. Drinking too much can depress sexual libido.)

● *Build in time to be with your partner without pressure*. If your idea of together time is shopping at Sainsbury's on a Saturday with a screaming baby in tow, it's time to think again. Many couples find that their personal time is characterised by interruptions or only happens when there is a task to be accomplished, with DIY taking top place in the 'pressured time' list. Pick a part of the day when you can be private, turn off the TV and other distractions, and just be together. Talk about what you want for the future, tell each other how much you mean to one another, and generally chill out.

● *Eliminate as much stress from your life as you can*. It's time to be honest about how much stress you are facing. Some stress is natural in everyone's life – deadlines at work, learning how to parent a baby, caring for a frail parent, for example

– but if you feel so stressed that you feel ill or exhausted all the time, you need to look for ways of removing stress from your life. Chronic stress is often caused by trying to put the needs of everyone else ahead of your own. Put your own hopes and wishes first more often and a great deal of stress will fall away. As Shakespeare has written, 'Self-love is not so vile a sin as self-denying'. Say 'no' more often and your blood pressure could improve overnight! (There is more on these issues in Chapters 4, Stress, and 6, Anger.)

How to feel good about sex

Anger, tiredness and anxiety are the most common causes of loss of desire. But there are other causes that trouble couples. As Val has pointed out in the first half of this chapter, what you learn about sex in childhood, or during adolescence, can have a profound influence on how you feel and think about sex. If you were told by your family, or just grew up feeling that sex is to be avoided, embarrassing or simply taboo, then you may find it hard to give your sexual desire full rein. This is rather like driving a car with the handbrake on. The car may go, but it will never reach its full potential. Eventually, the brakes will burn through and the car will stop. This is what happens to men and women who have mixed feelings about sex. They spend so much energy trying to hold on to, and make sense of, their emotions and physical responses that their capacity to enjoy sex with a loved partner becomes blunted.

Be in touch

If you recognise yourself as someone who feels ambivalent about wanting sex because you feel guilty, embarrassed or uncomfortable about sex here are some ideas to help you to be in touch with your natural sexual desire.

- Imagine yourself back in the situation where you feel sex was regarded as a dirty word. This might be as a child or teenager, in your family, at school or somewhere else. Think about what message you picked up (sometimes you may not have actively been told anything about sex, but simply absorbed a negative attitude). Now imagine yourself as an adult countering the attitude. For example, if you feel your family gave you the idea that sex was unpleasant, pretend you are asking the people you heard or believed made these remarks or held these attitudes why they feel this. If you engage in this imaginary debate for long enough you will probably discover that their attitudes come from their own poor sex education and personal prejudices.

- Think of all the arguments you can to allow you to let go of this way of behaving. It is also important to forgive them for any hurt they caused you, as they are only the product of the generations before them and may not have been able to break out of their own negative programming. It can help to write down your personal arguments – such as, 'sex with someone I love is a pleasure and helps us to feel closer to one another', 'I feel more confident and relaxed after love-making' or 'my mother was wrong to suggest that sex is mainly for men. Men and women can have equal pleasure from sex.' Now play back these positive statements when you notice negative thoughts about sex entering your mind. This will help your desire levels to rise.

- Allow yourself to enjoy sensual pleasures. If you have received negative messages about sex, it is likely that you have also learnt to damp down your pleasure at sensual stimulation. This is not just true for sexual issues. When was the last time you truly enjoyed the flavour of a good meal? Stroked a cat or dog and allowed yourself to feel the soft fur? Or sipped a cappuccino and let the gentle brush of the milky foam touch your lips? As an experiment, for one week allow yourself to wallow in all the sensual stimulation around you. Wear silky or soft underwear, use your best perfume or aftershave (even if you are only going to the office or supermarket), buy some scented flowers and put them all around your home and caress your skin with body lotion or shower gel. In other words, awaken your senses so that you gradually begin to feel more in touch with the pleasures of your body. Sexual desire doesn't just start in bed but needs input throughout the day if you are to be fully aware of your capacity to enjoy sex.

- Imagine yourself in your ideal sexual encounter. First of all, imagine the scene. Is it a country cottage in front of a roaring fire? By a mountain stream? At the seaside? Whatever you would like, try to see it in your head. Now fill in the details. What are you wearing (or not!)? Who are you with? What kind of love-making would you like – long and luxurious or quick and passionate? Try this exercise when you are able to be private and relaxed. Build up the picture until you can play it through your head easily. Now see yourself happy and relaxed in the middle of the scene, with no hang-ups or concerns. Try not to worry about whether you would really want this scenario in real life or not. This is a fantasy just for you so that you can understand that feeling turned on and interested in sex is possible for you, even if for the moment it is just in your head. In fact, you might never want some of the things that happen in your ideal location. This is just for fun. Eventually you may want to bring some elements of your fantasy into your real sex life – making love in front of the living room fire, for example, but for now just enjoy the mental image.

● Play this scenario through your head at least three times a week, altering anything you feel like changing. This is not to make you feel 'more sexy' (although it might) or just to provide you with a fantasy to use in love-making, but to help you see yourself as capable of sexual behaviour and feelings. Loss of desire often stems from a feeling that you have become 'sexless' in some way. Using this kind of 'play sex' helps to counteract this belief.

Seeking special help

Some people find that their sexual desire is cramped by difficult events from childhood. The most common of these is childhood abuse, by either a family member or someone else. About one in five people say they have experienced an inappropriate sexual event in childhood. This can prevent you enjoying sex, or create feelings of guilt when you do make love, so that sex becomes a minefield of emotional pain rather than a safe and loving pleasure.

But you should remember that whatever happened to you it was not your fault or responsibility. Even if you felt physical pleasure from the inappropriate touching, this does not mean that you invited the abuse. The adult who carried out the abuse, and anyone else involved, should have recognised your vulnerability and never allowed it to happen. If you have had this experience and want expert help, contact the National Association for People Abused in Childhood at 42 Curtain Road, London EC2A 3NH or at www.napac.org.uk.

Case Study catch up

Mike and Liz found that they were able to reconnect sexually by talking in depth about the effect of the affair. Liz also embarked on a regime of thinking more sexually. She created sexual images in her mind and created a range of fantasy situations. Mike saw that this helped Liz and he also allowed himself to think about sex in a more positive way. They put time aside for touching and cuddling, removing the sexual pressure on them that turned sex into a chore instead of a pleasure.

Your guide to touch

Touch is a crucial part of improving your desire for one another. Many couples who find sex boring or lacklustre do so because they stick to a sexual routine that rules out all the different elements of touch. So if you know you stick to just a few kinds of touch, consider using this guide to stimulating sensations, explained below. Start by using just one different kind of caress when you make love, building up to using a wider range over a period of a few months. Using a range of caresses on different parts of the body will improve your desire levels and enable you to feel closer to one another.

Stroking and caressing is usually carried out by using the flat of the hand in long strokes along the back, legs, breasts, stomach and shoulders. It is also arousing to have the face and hands stroked gently with light caresses. To improve the stimulating sensation of stroking further, loosely wrap a silk scarf around your hand before caressing your partner, or use a soft brush to caress his or her body gently. If you or your partner has long hair, trailing hair slowly over your partner's body can be highly arousing. Use your mouth and lips to caress your partner. Light kisses and soft licking over all parts of the body is highly stimulating. Stroking and caressing usually takes place at the start of love-making and can last from ten minutes to half an hour, or for as long as you both enjoy the sensation.

Massage

Body massage requires a firm touch during which you should use your hands not only to caress your partner's body but also to manipulate the muscles beneath the skin. Massage can also be used in a non-sexual setting to relax and ease tired muscles. During love-making, it can add to arousal because it helps you to relax and feel ready for sex. Ideally, you should take turns to massage each other. The back and shoulders are a good place to start, but upper arms and legs can benefit from massage techniques. Use good quality massage oil to help the hands slide over the skin without dragging. Massage is best given when there is plenty of time available to both of you and you need to turn off the stresses and strains of the day, and it is a good technique at the start of love-making: it can help you both to feel ready to enjoy the sexual experience. Massage is also a great way to say 'I love you' or to take you into your own special world, where the two of you can connect at an intimate level.

Kneading

Although a type of massage, kneading is stronger and firmer. Usually the hands are semi-clenched to allow use of the knuckles and fingers to press into the muscles – mostly on the back and buttocks. (Be careful: this technique can be painful if carried out incorrectly.) Used on the shoulders and neck it can help to relax knotted muscles. If you try this kind of massage, check out how your partner is feeling about it, and stop if they tell you they feel uncomfortable. Kneading can be a part of massage, or a separate form of touching, during the mid-stage of love-making. It should last not much more than ten minutes, as the sensation can be painful if carried on for too long.

Rubbing and circling

A rubbing action can often be particularly stimulating, especially if used with massage lotion or lubricant. Use the flat of the hand to rub in a circular fashion on the buttocks and thighs, breasts and back to produce a tingling sensation. Care should be taken not to press so hard that the rubbing becomes uncomfortable.

Rubbing is also extremely stimulating if used on the penis. A light but firm grip using the fingers around the penis is usually very arousing for men. Use a good quality lubricant to help your hand slide up and down the length of the penis without dragging the foreskin uncomfortably. Use plenty of lubricant – a silicone-based one is best – and gently circle the head of the penis, paying special attention to the frenulum (in uncircumcised men). Vary the length and speed of the strokes you use. Keep checking with your man that you are rubbing his penis in the way he finds arousing. Ask him to place his hand over yours to show you how he likes to be touched.

Circling is usually especially arousing for women. Once you are sure that the vaginal lips are well lubricated, run a finger along one side of them, around the clitoris and down the other side. Once fully stimulated, a circular motion around the area of the clitoris can be very exciting. Be wary of circling or rubbing directly on the clitoris, as this can be uncomfortable when a woman is highly aroused.

Rubbing and circling should be used during the mid to later stages of love-making and should last as long as both of you feel comfortable.

Tickling or teasing

Although a tickling or teasing touch can be annoying at other times, during love-making it can add to a stimulating experience if used carefully and with understanding. Intense stimulation, alternated with gentle fingertip touching and brushing of the genitals, can be extremely arousing. This approach can help to make love-making long-lasting. The variation between strong arousal and a softer touch can delay orgasm until both of you are ready to reach a climax.

Gentle tapping on the clitoral area or the head of the penis, or soft flicking with the tongue on the tip of the penis or clitoris, can be teasingly arousing. Stroking that is light and teasing can be arousing as it allows the person receiving the touch to want more intense and satisfying touching and arousal. Alternating firm stroking of the thighs and back with lighter, less intense, touching can improve sexual responsiveness and desire during love-making. Teasing and tickling should be part of mid and later stages of love-making and used for short periods of time (three to five minutes) according to your tastes.

Patting and smacking

Especially if concentrated on the buttocks and genital area, patting can be gently arousing. Soft rhythmic patting and light, firm squeezing of the whole vulval area can be enjoyable at the beginning of lovemaking. Some men also like their testicles patted, but this must be done gently to avoid any discomfort. Gently patting the clitoral area can be arousing because it introduces a teasing quality that many women enjoy in love-making. It can help if the woman holds the man's hand while he pats the vaginal lips and clitoris so that he understands how firm a touch she desires.

Smacking can also be arousing, but should be undertaken with caution and only with the agreement of your partner. Using the palm of the hand, men and women often enjoy having the buttocks smacked during sex. Three or four reasonably hard smacks to each buttock are probably enough for most people before the experience becomes painful rather than fun. Each of you should take the lead from your partner, and only carry on for as long as it seems enjoyable. It is also possible to use the flat back of a hairbrush, a ruler or a piece of stiff cardboard to smack a partner. But this must be done with care and consideration for their personal pain level. Patting can be used in the mid-stage of love-making, whereas smacking should be saved for late-stage arousal. At first, try gentle smacking, and stop when your partner indicates they have had enough. Most couples use gentle smacking as a fun extra rather than the focus of their love-making.

Licking and biting

The mouth is next only to the genital area in having many nerve endings that can supply and receive pleasure. Kissing, licking and biting can all be stimulating and arousing during sex play. Licking the thighs, buttocks, breasts and genitals can be extremely arousing. Slow, circling licking of the nipples is often intensely arousing. Try putting some cream or honey on to the nipple to boost the sensation. Intense licking along the length of the penis or vaginal lips is also highly arousing. The neck and ears are also particularly responsive when licked or kissed and can add to early arousal while your partner caresses other parts of the body.

Some couples also enjoy biting, although it is important to avoid breaking the skin as this can cause bleeding. This is important because some infections can be passed through contact with infected blood. Gentle biting or nibbling that does not break the skin is OK and can be arousing on the buttocks and neck. Love bites (sometimes called 'hickies') should be avoided, as there is a danger of infection from raising the blood to the skin, which then causes a bruise. (Blood can sometimes pass from the surface of the skin into the mouth during the giving of the love bite.)

Licking can be very intense during oral sex so the couple should discuss the length of time spent on this. Biting should be kept to a minimum, and only used in circumstances where you feel completely safe.

Pinching

Most people would say that pinching is not enjoyable in normal circumstances, but during sex pinching can be stimulating for some couples. You may find that light pinching of the nipples is arousing for some people, although others find it too painful to be stimulating. Pinching can also be stimulating on the buttocks or thighs. However, care should be taken to pinch areas of the body where there is plenty of flesh, as this will be more arousing and less painful than if pinching takes place on less fleshy areas, such as the wrists and shins. Pinching should be used as part of a much wider repertoire of touching, as it can be extremely uncomfortable if used without other kinds of caresses. Before attempting pinching, ask your partner how they feel about this kind of arousal.

Before you start, talk about how much pinching you think you can tolerate. Always start with gentle squeezes. Any prolonged pinching of nipples or flesh should be avoided – no more than a few seconds is sufficient – or the skin could be damaged, especially in the sensitive breast area.

Instant healing for loss of desire

- *Get back in touch with your body*. Caress your skin in the bath or with body oils and creams. Avoid criticising your shape or size. Instead, sink into the sensual messages your skin sends you.

- *Allow yourself to daydream about love-making and sexual imagery*. Even if this is not natural to you, remind yourself to think about sex at least a couple of times a day. For example, if you are looking at your garden or are in the park, imagine yourself making love on the warm grass. Remember, you don't have to actually want to do this in real life.

- *Check out your medication*. If you are taking antidepressants, the contraceptive pill or any other medication, ask your GP if it could be affecting your desire levels. A change of medicine could improve your sexual desire.

- *Question* if the messages your family, friends or school gave you about sex are valid. If they seem to repress your natural feelings, it is time to ask yourself if they really help you maintain a loving and sexual relationship.

● *Book a body massage*, an Indian head massage, a manicure or hairdressing appointment. In fact, do anything that means you allow another person to touch you in a way that helps you feel good about yourself. (But be wary of putting yourself in danger. Always check out a practitioner's training and qualifications.) Tune in to the pleasures of being touched so that you can take the feelings into love-making.

● *Masturbate two or three times a week*. Although you may not feel like doing this if your desire levels have shrunk, masturbating can actually awaken your sexual desire. If you are a woman, a vibrator could make a big difference to your response to sex. Go to www.emotionalbliss.co.uk for vibes designed especially for a woman.

● *Do things that encourage you to let go*. Visit a comedy club and laugh until you cry or dance wildly to a band you enjoy. Letting go, and feeling happy, can all lift your sexual desire.

KEY MESSAGE

In the long term, sexual desire has less to do with how you or your partner looks and much more to do with personal attitudes and behaviour. Thinking and behaving positively about sex can restore and rejuvenate desire.

CHAPTER 2

self-esteem

• •

The term, 'self-esteem', once favoured by psychologists, has seeped into everyday use. Editors of women's magazines are fond of features detailing 'Ten Ways to Boost Your Self-esteem', and practically every self-help manual advocates addressing issues of self-esteem if you want to lead an emotionally healthy and happy life.

This is one area where the media gets it right. Everyone should analyse at regular intervals how they feel about themselves. A few moments each day is probably enough when your life is ticking over satisfactorily.

Longer spells of introspection are best saved for times of crisis. If you feel you have a long-term problem with self-esteem after a deeply troubled childhood, or a seriously negative experience as an adult, consider talking to a counsellor or therapist with whom you feel comfortable. Their skills may help you make positive changes more swiftly than if you wrestle with overwhelming difficulties on your own.

You need confidence to make changes

Self-esteem matters because it plays a vital role in how you see yourself and your partnership. You can try making changes in your life, either alone or with a partner, but if you lack self-esteem it will be very hard to carry them through. This is principally because we are more motivated to make changes and handle the results when we feel good. Low self-esteem usually implies a lack of confidence, and few people are brave enough to instigate change when their confidence is in short supply.

What is self-esteem?

Self-esteem is a phrase bandied about by everyone from teenagers to the Prime Minister. The concept of high self-esteem usually has positive connotations, but for some people it reeks of arrogance, big-headedness and a tendency to put yourself forward at the expense of others. So let's clarify its meaning in the context of this chapter. Self-esteem in every-day life is about believing in your own effectiveness, in your ability to cope with life and being at ease with your self-image. It is about confidence – and few attributes are sexier than confidence.

The opposite of self-esteem

The opposite of self-esteem is being very self-critical, treating yourself harshly and not valuing your strengths and assets, preferring instead to focus on the negative. Obviously, this does you more harm than good. Believing self-critical thoughts – which are probably not even true – not only makes you feel bad but it also encourages you to act in self-defeating ways, creating a vicious circle of negative thoughts leading to destructive actions.

So if you think, 'I'm too fat to be sexy', the chances are you won't do anything that might make you feel sexy, like buy beautiful underwear, seduce your partner when they least expect it, or even accept compliments without assuming the other person doesn't mean what they say. It's easy to see how just one negative thought like this can lead to a downward spiral of bad feelings, which only reinforce your low self-esteem.

The differences between men and women

Some people believe that women value themselves by who they are and men value themselves by what they do. So if a woman's work is rewarding, and her family and friendships are functioning well, she will feel good.

A man, on the other hand, is more likely to feel positive about himself after winning promotion or buying the car of his dreams. Men tend to get more self-esteem as individuals from a successful sexual relationship too. This may be partly owing to taking masculine pride in keeping their sexual equipment regularly serviced.

A less obviously stereotypical explanation is that it is also because men often find it easier to demonstrate all aspects of their personality, including the so-called 'female' attributes of caring and tenderness, when they are in a physically and emo- tionally rewarding sexual relationship.

If you take this idea to its logical conclusion, it means that a good sexual relationship enables a man to feel more complete and in touch with all aspects of himself, thus rewarding him with better self-esteem.

The downside of this is that a man who is constantly rejected sexually by his partner can find his self-esteem seriously dented. By being unable to express himself sexually he may be losing out on access to other aspects of his nature, which literally makes him less of a man. (Of course, sexual rejection is tough for a woman too. But she is more likely to question her physical attractiveness in the first instance, rather than feel emotionally shut down as a result.)

Clearly these are broad generalisations, but they can be useful to bear in mind when it comes to understanding why your partner might be feeling a lack of self-esteem at any one time. This is because when one of you sinks in the self-esteem stakes, your 'couple self-esteem' will take a bit of a battering too. 'Couple self-esteem' is described later in this chapter, but it is worth remembering that how you both feel as individuals has a major impact on your couple relationship.

Of course, this may sound hugely obvious. However, you'd be surprised at the number of wives or husbands who will dismiss an aspect of their partner's life without thinking about the impact it is having on them. For example, saying something like 'Just because someone smashed your car, don't take it out on me' or 'Stop worrying about your sister and let's have sex' indicates that you aren't tackling things as a team. As a result your team spirit will start to dwindle, and your level of 'couple self-esteem', which is reflected in your sex life, will plummet.

Understanding sexual self-esteem

Sexual self-esteem is an extension of feeling sufficiently good about yourself so that you have the confidence to make your partner feel great too. It is about being comfortable with who you are and what you look like, which sounds easy, but, as most of us know, the journey to that place is not always straightforward.

The reason for this is that all around us we see evidence that would indicate that being happy with ourselves *as we are* is the last thing to which we should aspire. Advertising is based almost entirely on the idea that we are in some way deficient. We are not blonde enough, or attractive enough, and that without certain grooming and cleansing products no potential suitor could possibly find us attractive. If, on the other hand, we shave (either legs or faces, depending on gender), wash our hair with shampoo that practically promises an orgasm, squirt ourselves with powerful scent or aftershave, then we are guaranteed a trail of adoring followers who will want us above all else.

These are incredibly powerful messages, and we hear them constantly from a very young age. Western society, in particular, is awash with suggestions that in order to be sexually desirable women have to look a certain way. The usual template is that they must be slim, blonde, under 25, and accessorised with big breasts, high heels and a designer wardrobe.

'Slim' has become an accolade

Movies, magazines and television constantly reiterate a slim image and, frankly, as a result, it is almost impossible not to be seduced by it. If you ask any British man to describe what physical qualities he looks for in a woman, almost every one will say 'slim'. But when you ask them about women they have found attractive and dated in the past, it usually turns out that 'slim' can mean anything from a size eight to a size 16. Unfortunately, the word 'slim' has become an accolade, and as such it is frequently used to describe any attractive woman, whether or not she is actually slim.

In her excellent book *Fabulous Figures*, author Rachel Swift points out to the 90 per cent of women who go on weight-loss diets at some stage in their lives that men actually like variety. And that, surprise, surprise, there are some men who prefer plump women, some who like skinny women, but most of them are happy with someone in between whose personality they like and whose company they enjoy.

She also highlights the worrying statistic that fashion models are up to 19 per cent below the recommended weight for their height. One of the main diagnostic criteria for the crippling mental and physical illness anorexia nervosa is being more than 16 per cent below your recommended weight. So the majority of the role models featured in the magazines and commercials aimed at women in this country should probably be receiving help for a serious medical condition.

Rachel adds: 'Today, 80 per cent of the world's cultures consider plumpness desirable in women, 90 per cent of cultures consider large hips and thighs attractive. Yet women in the West, instead of celebrating their diversity and beauty, spend hours each day criticising their bodies and semi-starving themselves. Many now pay surgeons to cut them into shape.'

Fatness and fashion

Today, Marilyn Monroe at size 16 would be told by movie producers to get a personal trainer and lose a couple of stone, because fatness is a perception of fashion. But for many men there is no modern Hollywood heroine who outshines Marilyn's sex appeal.

Yet the message that there is only one way to be sexy, which is given out to women, is unrelenting and harsh. The way to begin to change your perspective, if you, like millions of us, have swallowed this myth, is to ask yourself a couple of pertinent questions.

Would my sex life be different if I was thin?

You may think you know the answer to this. You may imagine that you would easily attract men, you would feel confident naked and that you would be instantly multi-orgasmic. (Honestly, some people set such store by body weight that they truly believe they could lead a different life if only they were a couple of stones lighter.) The answer to this question is simple. Nothing changes when you lose weight unless you change. The corollary of this is that you can make changes in your sex life and gain sexual confidence *without* losing weight. The one thing you do need to lose, though, is your negative attitude to your body.

Would it be different if I had better self-esteem?'

Here you are on more useful territory. You can begin to imagine how you would like to be, what you will be doing and how you will be feeling. You might imagine feeling confident seducing your partner, knowing that they are weak with desire for you, and enjoying your sexual power over them (responsibly, of course!). Or you might imagine being attractive to strangers, and being able to flirt and have fun in a lighthearted and non-threatening way with people you find attractive.

The important thing is that whatever your image is of you having good sexual self-esteem, always keep it somewhere in your mind. Think about it at least once a day, preferably when you are feeling peaceful and relaxed. Just pay attention to those thoughts for a few minutes and then let them go. If you want to work harder at this and make the changes faster, write your thoughts down and keep your notes somewhere safe.

Four steps to start positive change

1. Pick out five things your like about yourself. Most people with low self-esteem about their self-image can hardly bring themselves actually to look at their bodies. So you can begin to change this pattern now by looking in the mirror and picking out five things that you like about yourself. These don't have to be particular facial characteristics, like your nose or your mouth (although they can be if you love your pert nose or your luscious lips). They can include shapes, curves or something about the way your body moves which gives you pleasure.

2. Then ask your partner, a female friend and your mother, or a close relative, to do the same for you. You may be astonished, and pleasantly gratified, by the physical things they like. And you'll be guaranteed that someone will remark with admiration on something that you may have barely noticed about yourself.

3. Resist the temptation to draw attention to what you perceive as your bad points, as in 'I hate my nose, it's HUGE', or 'my bum is saggier than a sackload of potatoes', and so on. It is a way of guaranteeing that people will definitely now notice what they have probably not noticed before.

4. Watch your body language, too. Often, when you try to cover up something, such as a spot on your cheek, you end up inadvertently drawing attention to it. There is no mysterious reason for this. It's simply because we tend to follow the focus of attention of whoever we are speaking to. If you are focusing on trying to hide one side of your face with a flap of hair that keeps resisting, for example, you can be guaranteed that whoever you are talking to will soon be transfixed by your attempts. Whereas if you simply greeted them with a sunny smile and concentrated on them, they'd never notice your zit, even if you feel it's the size of Wales.

For women in particular, lack of self-esteem leads them to focus on the physical attributes they like least. Although changing the way you think about a body you don't like can feel like trying to turn round an ocean liner in full steam, gradually you will be able to make changes that can profoundly affect the way you view yourself.

Do only beautiful people have great sex?

I hope it's not taken you more than a couple of seconds to reply 'no'. You could be forgiven for having to mull it over, though. Although it is clear that all the blessings that good genes and expensive cosmetic surgeons can bestow rarely keep celebrities in happy, sexually fulfilled, long-term relationships, we continue to be sold the myth that so-called beautiful people have a better time in bed.

This is partly because the only other people we see having sex are Hollywood and porn stars, and as a rule they seem to be good-looking and wildly enthusiastic about it. What we forget is that *they are pretending*. The minute the director shouts 'cut' they climb off each other, exchange pleasantries about the weather and go off to their dressing rooms and have a cup of tea on their own.

The fact that we are all duped by this into believing that you should look a certain way if you really want to let go in bed would be comical if it did not have such tragic repercussions. Thousands of women refuse to make love on top of their partners (denying themselves one of the most pleasurable positions for a woman) because they are worried he will see the size of their stomach, notice their stretch marks, or observe that their breasts are no longer as pert as they used to be.

This insecurity makes them want to make love with the lights out and undress in the dark. It mars the sexual satisfaction of thousands of couples. So I would like to address the next sentence to women, and trail it in letters 12 metres (40 feet) high from an aircraft across the sky:

Rational men do not care about physical perfection

If a man loves you, I promise you he will be pretty much blind to what you perceive as your defects. And if he doesn't love you, he will still be pretty damn grateful that you are in bed with him in the first place. A man who makes you feel bad about your body does not deserve the privilege of a kiss from you, let alone sex.

Ask any man what he would prefer in a lover: physical perfection or enthusiasm, 99 per cent will reply 'enthusiasm', and the 1 per cent who reply 'physical perfection' are best avoided.

If you are still unconvinced that this is the case, try something different next time you make love with your partner. Buy some massage oil and take it in turns to give each other a gentle massage. Play some gentle background music, and, as you massage, whisper something you love or like about your partner's body in their ear. It can be anything from the shape of their neck to a delicate fold of skin behind their knees. If you are the recipient, don't argue or say 'how on earth could you like that?' Just accept the compliments and the massage and be prepared to return the favour.

Too old to have great sex?

So how old is too old to have great sex? Seventy? Eighty? Ninety? If you are reeling in horror at the thought of what people get up to in retirement homes, give yourself a stern telling off and remind yourself that 'old' is always 15 years older than you – *no matter what your age*. Our uncomfortable response to the idea of sex and the elderly is partly linked to the idea of our parents having sex and also takes us back to my *bête noire* of Hollywood and porn films, when you rarely see anyone over the age of 40 experiencing sexual desire. This is a pernicious misrepresentation of reality and can fuel uncomfortable feelings in people as they grow older, damaging their self-esteem as lovers.

You can be a good lover at 50, a great one at 60 and a fantastic one at 70 and beyond. Good sex has very little to do with physical perfection. It is about fun and sharing – neither of which is prohibited as you grow older. For some people it is about an emotional and even spiritual connection that deepens with the passing years.

The best sex

When we can express who we truly are with another person we will enjoy the best sex, and that rarely happens in the first flush of youth (often because when we are young, we don't yet know who we truly are). Maturity brings self-awareness and, hopefully, self-acceptance. These are two qualities that should boost your self-esteem as a lover, no matter what your age.

Keep your self-esteem high

Sexual self-esteem is crucial to most satisfying intimate relationships. As Val has written, feeling low about your body or some other aspect of your life can put a damper on your sex life. If you feel bad about yourself, or your life in general, it can be very difficult to let go and enjoy sex with your partner. Here is Wesley and Maria's story. As you read about their concerns with self-esteem, look for aspects of their account that you identify with.

CASE STUDY . . . .

Wesley and Maria

Wesley and Maria, both aged 28, have lived together for three years. They met through friends and clicked almost immediately. They moved in to Maria's flat within four months of meeting and feel very close to one another. The only problem they have is Maria's attitude to her body. Maria feels she has fat thighs and a large bottom. This means that whenever she and Wesley make love she avoids showing her thighs and bottom. She keeps very still during sex and usually tries to keep the duvet over her legs. Wesley is mystified by this behaviour. He likes Maria's figure and regards her curves as immensely attractive. He felt this from the start of the relationship and although he has frequently told Maria how lovely she is, she finds it almost impossible to believe him.

Maria comes from a large family with five brothers. As she reached puberty her brothers began to tease her about her figure, telling her she was overweight and that her 'bum was huge'. In her teens, she tried to ignore these remarks. During this time, she often cried herself to sleep, because she believed she was ugly. Maria has had several boyfriends but has never felt comfortable about sex because she always feared they privately thought her body was not as attractive as it should be. She knows she loves Wesley, but also feels anxious that he is 'just being nice' when he says she is sexy and beautiful.

Maria and Wesley do argue about sex but Maria usually ends up in tears, which causes Wesley to back off, as he hates upsetting her. He would also like more adventurous sex – different sexual positions and with Maria wanting to caress him more willingly, for example – but he fears this is never going to happen while Maria feels as badly about her body as she does. They feel stuck in a sexual impasse that Wesley does not know how to break and that Maria is afraid to investigate.

. . . .

Lack of sexual self-esteem can cause sex to become routine and bound by invisible rules that the couple may never fully under-stand. Not all these problems stem from body image, as in Maria's case, but can originate in a fear of certain sexual practices, general feelings of not being 'good enough' or previous criticism of your sexual prowess by your partner or a previous partner. Challenging these is not always easy, but if you want to build self and couple esteem, you may need to look these issues squarely in the eye.

Improving body self-esteem

Many people identify this issue as a problem in love-making. They fear that their body does not match the images they see in adver-tising or in films, or that their body has changed so much over the years (got fatter, saggier, wrinklier, and so on) that it is somehow not acceptable to their partner. While it is important to be body aware from a health point of view, the idea that your body is not attractive to your partner because (if you are a woman) you have small breasts or big thighs, or (if you are a man) lack muscular arms, is clearly not reflected in the population. Just think of the couples of every shape and size you see walking down the street. If physical perfection was the only criteria for couples building a sexual relationship the birth rate would drop to nil in a very few years! Body shape is also subject to the vagaries of fashion. If you were a plump woman during the Twiggy era, or a thin woman in Rubens's pictures, you would have been worrying about completely opposite issues: how to get thinner or fatter. Yet both of these body shapes were considered perfectly acceptable by the fashion of the time. The crucial thing here is to understand that you need to feel comfortable with your own body, whatever its shape and whichever era you live in. Natural body shape is neutral. It is fashion and social conditioning that determines what we do with our bodies. How else can you explain women of today having breast implants and women of the 1920s binding their breasts to be as flat-chested as possible?

The key to body esteem is to value and honour your body for how it is today – not how you think it ought to be in six months after you have joined a gym or how it was ten years ago when you were two stone lighter.

Getting in touch with your body

Try this exercise to get you started on valuing your body as it is rather than how you wish it was:

> Run yourself a warm bath. (You could also do this exercise in the shower if you do not have a bath.) Make sure you use your favourite oil, lotion, or soap. Lay back (or stand comfortably if you are in the shower) and close your eyes.

Now, using the lather in the bath or shower, stroke your body. Allow yourself to feel the softness of your skin, silky hair, weight of your breasts and shape of your arms and legs. Use your hands to explore your body gently as if you were encountering it for the first time. Include your neck and face, as these are often neglected areas of sensual pleasure.

If you find that negative thoughts intrude ('I'm too fat', 'I wish my breasts/pecs were larger/smaller', 'My last boyfriend/ girlfriend criticised my body') replace the thoughts with 'My skin is soft and smooth', 'I love the curve of my back' and 'I feel relaxed and warm'.

This can take some practice. If you have spent the last 20 or 30 years telling yourself you are flawed and unattractive, one bath will not counter this toxic input. You need to do this every time you bathe or shower. Gradually you will feel better about your body as you reprogramme your thinking.

An advanced level of this exercise is to find a private place and time when you can be uninterrupted:

Lay a towel on your bed to protect your bed linen, and remove your clothes. Lay on the towel and, using body lotion or oil, gradually caress all of your body with the lotion. As you do this, enjoy the sensations of your skin texture and body shape.

Try to relax into the sensual experience rather than doing a lot of mind work. As you smooth yourself, allow the good feelings to replace any negative emotions.

If you feel sexually aroused during this exercise, avoid masturbating. Instead, notice the feelings you experience and enjoy their effect on you, letting go of the desire to have an orgasm.

When you have stroked every part of your body, cover

yourself with a towel, duvet, or sheet and spend 15 minutes relaxing. Breathe slowly and deeply to aid relaxation. A useful guide is to breathe in to a count of three, hold the breath for a count of three, and release the breath slowly, through the mouth, to a count of three. Meditation uses this kind of breathing because it aids stress reduction. As you breathe in this way, think of the pleasurable sensations you have enjoyed as you caressed yourself.

The aim of these exercises is to help you realise that your body can be a source of great pleasure, regardless of its shape and size. When you make love, the shape of your body is much less important than the tactile responses of your skin. The way your skin responds to touch, and how you respond to touching your partner, is what counts, not whether the shape of your body or theirs is fashionable or not. Of course, we all fancy different things about people – tall, short, blonde, brunette, skinny, plump, black or white – but, essentially, if you care about the person you are with, it is the messages from your skin that counts. If you have personal body confidence and esteem, your shape and size will be irrelevant. This will communicate itself to your partner and they will feel thrilled at your warmth and openness, and certainly not worried about your thighs or chest size.

Couple self-esteem

How do you feel about your relationship? Does it feel like a wet January day or a sunny June afternoon? If your relationship feels grey and miserable then it should be no surprise that your sex life feels depressed and lacking in sparkle. Low couple esteem causes a variety of problems. Money worries, overwork, and lack of time together, childcare issues and concerns about health can all lead to you feeling that sex is lacklustre and boring. But a satisfying intimate life can actually help you survive the problems you encounter in everyday life. Sex can be bonding, life affirming, emotionally satisfying and joyful. Even if the credit card is up to the limit, sex is free and great for your sense of couple esteem! I am not suggesting you use sex to pretend you do not have any problems; rather that you see it as a way of keeping you focused on your love for one another and a 'together we can do anything' attitude.

Here are some ways to help you improve intimacy and build a sense of togetherness:

- **Examine when you are trying to make love or be close to one another.** Are you putting everything else before your sex life? If you find you fall into bed at the end of a very long day and think 'I suppose we ought to have sex now' you are bound to feel that the experience is less than you hoped. You will be tired, distracted by the events of the day and probably dying to get to sleep – a sure recipe for unsatisfying sex. Try going to bed earlier, putting time aside for love-making at other times (such as lazy weekend lie-ins) and making the best use of time when you can be alone; for example, when the kids are staying with a friend and you have the house to yourself. It's tempting to think that any non-work time should be used in other activities such as DIY, visiting friends or shopping. If you put these before sex then don't be surprised if sex seems very much like a 'bottom of the list' experience.

- **Tell each other what you find attractive about one another.** Cuddle up on the sofa or lie on the bed together and take it in turns to say what you find sexy and attractive about your partner. For example, say, 'I love the way your nose crinkles up

when you smile', 'I can never see the nape of your neck without wanting to kiss it', or 'I love your curvy bum.' Think about
every part of the body as well as just those in the erogenous
zones. Hands, faces and feet are often neglected areas for
praise. Spend at least half an hour doing this. Kiss and cuddle
if you would like to. Avoid making love unless and until you
have found ten complimentary things to say about each other.
You could end this exercise with just a cuddle rather than sex,
but if you go on to make love continue to use your compliments during love-making. You can also praise your partner
when they do something that really turns you on. For example, 'I love it when you stroke me there' or 'If you hold me this
way it feels great'.

- *Lengthen the time you spend on love-making.* Most unsatisfying sex and low sexual esteem is the result of fast,
unsatisfying sex (except for those passionate moments when
you just cannot wait to get to each other!). You can even make
a pact that you will not attempt intercourse until you have
spent at least half an hour in arousing one another. Use your
hands, mouth, and lips to stimulate your partner and ask for
the same in return. Although a man can reach orgasm more
quickly than a woman, both men and women report the
pleasure they share in extended mutual stimulation. If you
feel you are getting close to climax by this kind of arousal
alone, just rest for a few minutes until the peak of arousal dies
away a little. Then resume stimulation. This will not only
extend your love-making, but also give you both a more
intense orgasm because of the degree of excitement you will
have built up.

- *Outside of love-making, tell each other how important you
are to one another.* For example, say, 'You are so important to

me', 'You really turn me on when we make love' and 'Your body is so erotic.' It is surprising that many couples ignore this simple way of boosting couple esteem. This is rather like living in an emotional desert where you are always hoping for an oasis to appear. If you talk about sex only at the moment of climbing into bed together it can also leave you both feeling that one or both of you is only being complimentary because they 'just want sex', even if they really mean what they are saying. So sex becomes an area for dissent instead of a place of regeneration in the relationship.

A guide to kissing

You're probably reading this and wondering how kissing fits into self-esteem. Surprisingly, it has an important part to play in committed relationships, which is often overlooked. Once a relationship is established, couples often give up the passionate kissing that they did so easily when they first got together. This is a real shame because a loving kiss can boost your self-esteem immediately. If your partner rushes home from work, grabs you at the front door, kisses you with real feeling and says, 'I've been longing to do that all day', your self-esteem will soar. Kissing also confirms the closeness of your relationship, allowing you to feel good about your couple esteem. Here are some tips and reminders to help you get the most from kissing:

● ***Always make sure your mouth and teeth are clean.*** Kissing someone with garlic breath is not pleasant. Clean your teeth regularly, use a mouthwash and visit your dentist for regular check-ups to keep your breath smelling fresh. Sometimes bad breath (halitosis) is caused by stomach or gut problems. Try taking a probiotic yogurt first thing in the morning and drink plenty of water to keep your gut healthy. Recurrent halitosis should be checked out by your GP.

- *Have you given up the long, lingering kiss in favour of the tight-lipped peck?* Do you avoid kissing during love-making? Try the following. As you place your lips against your partner's, consciously relax them. Imagine the muscles around your mouth becoming soft and pliant. Avoid rushing into French kissing (tongues in each other's mouths). Instead, gently brush your lips against his or hers. Press your lips against your partner's so the moist inner side of your lip touches theirs. Now, let your lips move slowly from side to side, lapping against their lips. It can feel very sexy to place your hands under your partner's hair or hold their head lightly in your hand. Women particularly like this technique, as it can feel relaxing to have their partner take control of the kiss, as well as signalling 'I find you so sexy I want to keep you here'. Once you have enjoyed this phase, then you can use your tongue. Never forcefully push your tongue into your partner's mouth. Gradually introduce your tongue by moving it luxuriously in and out. When you feel confident, hold your partner close to you, and alternate kissing with tongues to kissing without tongues.

- *Once you have reinvigorated your kissing*, try kissing your partner's neck and ear lobes during a passionate kiss. Little nibbles and soft kisses in these areas are highly arousing and often overlooked.

- *As your confidence grows* you can experiment a little. If you have ever kissed on a beach, particularly when a breeze is blowing, you will know how sexy kissing can be when lips are salty. You can put a little salt on your lips with a damp finger to remind you of kisses on the beach (but be sparing or you will taste like a fish and chip supper!). If you like this, try a dusting of icing sugar, cocoa powder or fruit juice.

- *For advanced kissing*, and probably most arousing during love-making itself, use ice cubes, chocolate or the alcoholic spirit of your choice. Place a small piece of ice (an ice chip is better than a whole cube) in your mouth, pass it to your partner in a kiss, encouraging them to return it to you until it melts. The combination of cold ice, soft mouth, and warm lips can be highly erotic. Try the same thing with a small piece of chocolate until it vanishes, or a mouthful of your favourite spirit (Bailey's or whisky works well, but check out what your partner likes first). Pass the liquid between you until you swallow it. The taste will linger on your and your partner's lips, giving you both a thrill as you kiss each other again.

- *Most people close their eyes when they kiss*, but occasionally try kissing with your eyes open, looking at one another. Not everyone enjoys this, but it can add a frisson of naughtiness to kissing. 'Eye locking' during a kiss can also feel adventurous and as if you are desperate to hold on to each other – which of course you are!

- *Play a kissing game.* Take it in turns to kiss a part of each other. Erotic and overlooked areas are the fingers and toes, ear lobes, backs of knees and armpits. Offer soft, butterfly-like kisses or nibbling-like nips, or take your partner's fingers into your mouth one by one, slowly releasing them as you remove them from your mouth. You may wish to place an embargo on the sexual organs so you can get to know each other's parts of the body.

How to practise Kegel exercises

Many women worry about whether their vagina is tight enough and this can affect their self-esteem. The vagina is not an open tunnel, but a soft tube that gradually lengthens and widens during arousal. It is shaped like an upside down wine bottle, with the most sensitive section at the entrance. Stretching of the vagina occurs naturally during childbirth, and although it may be a little wider after childbirth, the idea that it somehow gapes open so that stimulation to the penis declines is a myth. What can happen, however, is that the muscles (called the pubococcygeus, or PC, muscles) that run in a hammock shape from the pubic bone at the front of the pelvis to the anus lose their tone. These muscles are like any other muscle in the body. If they are not used, or experience a trauma such as childbirth, they need to be built up. Creating toned PC muscles can help improve your sexual pleasure and, in some women, give them more intense orgasms.

The best way to start is to clench these muscles by imagining you are trying to stop a flow of urine. You can experiment with this on the toilet, but don't keep doing this as it is not good for your bladder function. Once you have found the muscles you need to work on, do these muscle clenches throughout the day. Contract the muscle, hold it for three seconds and then release. Do this in sets of ten throughout the day. Nobody need know you are exercising in this way. When you have mastered this method, try quick squeezes and releases several times a day. You will need to keep this up for six to eight weeks to see a difference.

You can also exercise these muscles by squeezing your partner's penis when he is in your vagina. Most men find this incredibly erotic, and some women perfect the art so that they learn to 'milk' his penis to orgasm. This takes a lot of practice, and well-toned PC muscles, but there is no reason why you should not aim for this nirvana of PC exercises!

Men can also try Kegel exercises. They should contract the muscles in the anus and between the legs. Some men report it helps to give their erect penis a more 'standing out' effect, which boosts their sexual self-esteem.

Kegel exercises are also good for bladder control, so if you are a woman who has a problem with losing small amounts of urine when you reach orgasm, these exercises can help to prevent this. Expelling a small amount of urine during orgasm is very common and happens because the PC muscles relax and tighten during the waves of pleasure that orgasm creates. If this worries you, place a towel on the bed and keep some tissues to hand. It is unlikely that your partner would even notice this happening, especially if you don't need to use a condom and his ejaculate also spills out of the vagina after love-making. Try not to worry about it because anxiety will make it much more likely to happen. If you lose a lot of urine, or experience pain at the same time, see your GP for help.

When self-esteem feels under attack

For some individuals, self-esteem can feel very low indeed, even though they are in a committed relationship. This is because they feel that their partner is actively attacking their sense of sexual self-esteem. The reasons why this happens can be complex but they tend to be mainly owing to a desire to control a partner in some way. For example, the man who tells his wife she is unattractive, or rubbish at sex, might be trying to stop her exploring her sexuality – and finding out that it is he that lacks sexual technique. Alternatively, the woman who tells her husband that no other woman would have him might be afraid of him leaving her. There is more about this subject in Chapter 5 (Power Games), but if someone is trying to dent your self-esteem by belittling you, the relationship needs serious attention. True love means wanting the best for your partner and supporting their self-confidence, not knocking him or her down until they feel bad about themselves. Never accept a partner's negative view at face value. Whatever their opinion, you deserve care and concern for your feelings and ideas. Believe in yourself and tell them how you feel about their attitude. There is no room for low self-esteem in the bedroom.

Case Study catch up

Maria and Wesley found that their problems about Maria's low self-esteem were helped by talking about what they enjoyed in sex outside of love-making. They also spent some evenings telling each other what they found attractive about one another. Maria found she relaxed more and was able to appreciate what Wesley had been trying to tell her – that she was an attractive woman.

Quick boosts for sexual self-esteem

- **Put time aside for love-making** in the same way you put time aside to play or watch sport, visit friends, or go shopping. If it helps, mark your diary with evenings or other times when you can be together without interruptions.

- *Use items around the home to improve your sexual experience.* Wrap a silk scarf around your hands to caress your partner. Drape a necklace chain between your hands and gently trickle it over your partner's body. Ask them to do the same for you. Make love on a fur rug or silk sheet. Offer to towel-dry your partner after their bath or shower, or soap them with a sponge or your hands while they bathe. Look for the sensuous opportunities in ordinary things in your home.

- *Slow sex down.* Most people have problems with sex because they rush to the end. Think of it as a journey where you enjoy the view on the way as well as the destination. Agree a 'love pact' of at least half an hour of arousal and caressing before attempting intercourse. Allow yourself to get close to orgasm, stop for a few minutes and then resume arousal. If you do this three or four times during your love play your orgasm will be extremely intense.

- *Pamper yourself.* This does not mean spending money on expensive treats. Instead, allow yourself relaxation and fun time. See yourself as worthy of care and concern rather than a machine that must be run into the ground.

- *Don't draw your sense of yourself from what other people tell you.* Concentrate on building up your own sense of self-worth. For example, tell yourself how attractive you are rather than how fat/wrinkly/unkempt you are.

- *Enjoy your body.* Simple grooming such as regular haircuts, pleasant scent and clothes you feel confident in will help you to feel your body is a source of pleasure rather than something that must be denied and mistreated. Eat sensibly and take exercise that makes you feel good. Over- or under-eating, lack of exercise or punishing your body with too much exercise do not honour your body and can make you hate yourself rather than love who you are.

● *Live in the now.* Wishing things could be different in the future, or yearning for the past, mean you miss the pleasures you could have today. Seize the moment and live for those things that make you happy or fulfilled.

KEY MESSAGE

Self-esteem begins in the head, not in the body. Value yourself, your achievements, and your body. Your sex life will improve overnight.

CHAPTER 3

parenting

. . . .

Mums and dads aren't sexy. Good parents may make you feel secure, be a source of comfort and support, and cheer you up when you are down, but part of the physical and emotional deal of family life is that as we grow up we turn off our sexual feelings towards our parents.

As a species, humans are programmed to do this as part of our physical survival, which is one of the reasons why incest is taboo in practically all societies. And when this taboo is broken, as survivors of parental sexual abuse know, lives can be shattered in its wake.

It is a sad irony that the desire to stay together and create a family, which is often awakened by an intense physical attraction between a couple, becomes the very thing that eventually extinguishes sexual desire between them. Countless couples enjoy perfectly happy sex lives before they marry, for example, only to discover that the marriage that they thought would bring them the added bonus of security and commitment seems to be strangling their sex life.

Is it better *not* to settle down?

So does this mean that if you want a good sex life, it is better not to settle down? The answer to this is a resounding NO. It is not the commitment itself that is to blame for the change in sexual desire, it is the associations and roles that couples adopt, either consciously, or more frequently unconsciously, when they marry or move into a serious, long-term relationship.

Most often, this turning point is reached when you decide to have a baby. In *Heartburn*, the dramatised story of Hollywood screenwriter Nora Ephron's marriage break-up, she reflects: 'A child is a grenade. When you have a baby, you set off an explosion in your marriage, and when the dust settles, your marriage is different from what it was. Not better, necessarily, not worse, necessarily; but different.'

The physical demands a small child imposes on a couple can't be underestimated: sleepless nights, a fundamental change in working patterns and routine (unless you employ professional help, and even that will precipitate shifts in lifestyle), an alteration to finances, and above all, the knowledge that you are no longer able to do as you please. It is small wonder that in the year after the first baby arrives, 70 per cent of wives experience a serious drop in their level of marital satisfaction. (Husbands usually experience an equivalent decline slightly later, as a reaction to their wives' unhappiness.)

Becoming mum and dad

Considerable as these stresses are, they are widely known and in some ways you can prepare yourself for them. What most of us aren't aware of, though, is an equally significant shift that happens inside us. This is the psychological stress of taking on new roles as mum and dad.

When we become parents we can become acutely aware of the messages we got from our own parents, even if in the time between leaving home and forming a long-term, adult relationship ourselves we spent every moment repudiating every word of homespun wisdom they delivered. You may no longer wear a vest, you may stay out to all hours and treat your home like a hotel, but the minute you have a child of your own, those parental voices will be echoing inside your head whether you like it or not.

If you add to this the fact that many people unconsciously, or even consciously, choose a marriage partner who reminds them of a parent, it is small wonder that it can become difficult to continue to see that person as a sexual being and to have sexual feelings for them.

Exit wild sex queen

The arrival of a baby is physical proof of our new status as a mother or father and surprisingly often this means that we unconsciously recategorise our partner accordingly. So the wild sex queen exits stage right and re-enters as a mum in a baggy tracksuit, breastfeeding a tiny baby. Sexually speaking, this can have a profound effect on both partners.

The woman may feel delighted with her new role, or she may feel dowdy, exhausted and not remotely sexual. Her partner may see the breasts which previously brought him so much pleasure fulfilling their other purpose as providers of food, and it may leave him feeling proud or confused, or irrationally jealous – or even a combination of all three.

His confusion may have arisen as soon as his partner found out she was pregnant. Some men struggle with the well-documented Madonna/whore complex: when they see women as pure and unsullied mothers or sexual creatures, but never both. In this instance, a man will find that when his partner transforms herself into the mother of his unborn child, it changes his instincts towards her and alters the relationship from the moment the dye in the pregnancy testing kit turns blue.

Great sex after the arrival of a baby

So to continue (or even to start) having great sex after the arrival of a baby, you need to tackle this challenge on two fronts. The first is to organise yourselves so that you can continue to function as a couple, as well as a family. And the second, which is a corollary to the first, is to ensure that you continue to label each other as lovers, friends and playmates, and not just as mum and dad.

Agony aunts are fond of saying that the best thing you can do for your children is to put your marriage first, and they are right. In the most obvious sense, this does mean getting a babysitter and going out together. It also means not talking about your children for the entire evening when you do go out, but relating to each other in the way you did before you were parents – sharing jokes that no one else knows, exchanging kisses in a side street, and talking about your hopes and dreams for the future.

It also means caring for your child or your children as *a couple*. Often it is the woman who takes maternity leave from work, or who gives up her job when the baby arrives, and automatically she assumes the greater share of caring for the baby. While this may make sense on one level, if her partner is not given an important role in looking after his child as well, he will easily drift into the background and sooner or later he will begin to feel overlooked and resent his loss of importance in her eyes.

Why some men have affairs

Some men are tempted into affairs shortly after their wives have a baby, and although women are inclined to blame themselves for not being attractive any more, or to dismiss their partners as bastards if they find out, the simple truth is often that the man is missing out on the attention he used to receive from his partner.

Women reason that their partner is an adult – of course he can cope without her attention. Men, however, frequently feel alienated and lonely as they observe the single-minded, all-consuming love and care devoted by some women to their new babies.

Some women, too, are susceptible to affairs with the arrival of a baby. If a woman feels unsupported by her partner and consumed by the demands of a young child, a man who flatters her with attention and reminds her that she is a sexual being beyond the world of sandpits and nappies can be an enticing port of call.

A lot of women become impatient with dads when they clumsily try to feed a baby or get the temperature of the bath wrong. Tempted as she may be to whisk the baby back to her confident, capable hands, a woman who wants to keep her couple relationship alive knows that dads need to get involved at the earliest stages in order to bond with their offspring and not resent them.

A man has to accept that he will never get his wife back exactly as she was before she became a mother. But if he follows her enthusiastically into parenthood, and if they can pull off the trick of keeping their couple relationship alive as well, so that instead of swapping one role for another they add another dimension to themselves, the experience of parenting can allow both of them to become emotionally richer individuals.

Interestingly, statistics have shown that women who are responsible for more than 80 per cent of parenting long term are more likely to instigate divorce, sometimes reasoning that as they are practically a single parent anyway they would do better on their own.

Viewing her partner as a child

In these circumstances, the relationship often breaks down because the woman views her partner almost as another child she has to take care of. And if a man offers very little support to her in looking after the family, but expects attention and care from her nevertheless, then you can understand her point of view.

On the other hand, some women fall into the trap of treating their husbands like children and then complaining when they don't act like men. If a man doesn't know how the washing machine works and can't organise a meal, for example, I'd say he is in a dangerously dependent – or childlike – state.

There are, of course, couples that are happy with very clear divisions of labour that entail a man going out to work and a woman staying at home to run the house and take care of the children; the kind of set-up that operated widely a generation or so ago when it was automatically assumed that a woman would stop working outside the home if she had a family. And if both you and your partner are perfectly content with this arrangement, then you don't have a problem.

When both partners work

Difficulties arise when assumptions are made about roles, again often unconsciously, and it turns out that one or both parties resent what's going on. Bearing in mind that in 67 per cent of relationships now both partners work, it's not rocket science to see that domestic arrangements should shift accordingly. But the imprints we receive when we are young are immensely powerful, and it's astonishing how many couples slip into trying to replicate their parents' traditional roles, even though their own circumstances are very different.

This neatly leads us back to the idea of what author Dagmar O'Connor calls learning to 'unMummy' and 'unDaddy' your-selves in order to rekindle or kick-start your sex life. In her bestselling book *How to Make Love to the Same Person for the Rest of Your Life*, she explains:

The process of 'UnMummying' our wives and 'UnDaddying' our husbands begins in our minds, where the confusion started: first, it would be foolish to try to convince ourselves that we are going to totally exclude our 'Mummying' and 'Daddying' roles from our relationship. These roles, after all, are part of the reason we got married in the first place: for the comfort and security it affords us. But we must see that being a 'maternal comfort' to our husband is only *one* of the roles we can play – *one of many*. And it does not have to exclude other roles – the role of friend, co-adventurer, and *lover*. Mature men and women can learn to make the transition from 'Mummy' or 'Daddy' to 'Lover' without having to feel confused or guilty.

From 'mummy and daddy' to red-hot lovers

So how do you switch from being mummy and daddy to red-hot lovers – or even reasonably warm lovers – bearing in mind that our unconscious minds may have turned us into our parents without us even realising? The first step is to acknowledge that when you realise something about a previously unconscious thought process, the very process of thinking about it in your conscious mind means that you are now capable of doing something about it.

So a woman who was once attracted by the boyish charm of her husband can begin to understand why she finds his childlike behaviour so irritating now he is a father. If she accepts that he is failing to live up to the 'daddy' role she now has allotted him in her mind's eye, she can rethink her attitude, and even explain how she now needs some more mature behaviour in certain areas.

And if she can still relish the energy and eagerness that she previously enjoyed in her husband, she has a much greater chance of still finding him physically attractive, as he won't have morphed entirely into the unsexy figure of 'dad'.

Don't shut down

When a couple do see each other solely as mum and dad, their body language changes accordingly. They tend to give each other chaste hugs and kisses; the sort that you offer other family members. It is as though they shut down on the idea that affection can lead to sex. Dagmar O'Connor suggests that in order to become sexual again, you need to break this self-imposed physical barrier between you deliberately.

She says: 'It is a question of allowing ourselves to switch the focus, of catching ourselves before we automatically turn off. Try to remember that this hug, this kiss is *exactly the same physical act* which once made us delirious with sexual excitement; the *act* has not changed, only what we allow ourselves to feel has.'

So, as you embrace your partner, instead of cutting off at the point that you might with a child or a friend, deliberately choose to keep the embrace going and introduce a sexual element to it. If this feels awkward because it is a conscious choice rather than a spontaneous act, don't be put off. What you are doing is something very positive. And that is making a deliberate decision to keep your sexual relationship alive.

Your social life

Becoming parents can create a serious slump in your social life, as couples find that opportunities to pop out for a meal or a trip to the cinema now depend on handing over the care of their precious infant to granny or the teenager next door. In the early days of parenthood, when you are both feeling tired, this can seem like too much trouble, and it's easier to pick up a video and ring for a pizza.

While this may be a satisfactory solution in the short term, many couples simply lose the knack of socialising outside the home together. This can dent your relationship with each other in several ways. Perhaps most critically, it narrows your horizon to the end of your garden, and home itself is not an intrinsically sexy place. Sexual stimulation is not just a matter of pressing the right buttons physically. Your minds need to spark off each other too, and too much domesticity can smother fun and flirty behaviour towards each other.

If you are at home, surrounded by children's paraphernalia, the chances are your conversation will be mostly confined to talking about the visit from the washing machine repairman and the children's dental appointments. You don't have to spend a fortune on an expensive meal out or a weekend away (although saving up for both usually pays dividends), just a walk in the park and an ice cream on a sunny day will suffice, as long as you take an interest in each other.

Even if you are wildly successful at getting a social life after parenthood, you'll probably find that home is still the primary place for love-making, and if you have children there is nothing more of a desire-dampener midway through sex than a small person padding into the room, requesting a drink of water.

Fit a lock to your bedroom door

The simple answer to this is to *fit a lock to your bedroom door*. This will guarantee you some private space and it won't harm your children in any way. In fact, many psychologists would argue that if you make it plain to your children that you need time together as a couple, that message will help them build their own adult relationships. Even teenagers, who may be hugely embarrassed by the fact that you spend time together behind a locked door, will at least get the signal that it's OK for Mum and Dad to make love. And who knows? It may result in them growing into adult family relationships where they don't have to consciously 'unMummy' and 'unDaddy' each other.

'Empty-nest' syndrome

Maintaining your identity as a couple also means that when your children leave home, as they invariably will, you'll be able to accept the fact that they are forging their own paths without you much more easily. I find the term 'empty-nest syndrome' faintly derogatory, perhaps because it implies that a bird-brained parent (and it's a term usually applied to mothers) is failing to cope. But there is no doubting the trauma that both parents can experience as their youngest child leaves.

For women this often occurs around the time of the menopause, and there are some couples who are either consciously or unconsciously awkward about making love for pleasure, with no element of procreation involved. This may be rooted in a religious upbringing, or it may be an unspoken attitude that nevertheless circumscribes a couple's attitude towards each other.

If you believe this and you also believe that God designed the human form, it may help to know that a woman's clitoris serves no reproductive use at all. It is designed purely and utterly to bring her pleasure. Which suggests that making love and experiencing pleasure aren't necessarily linked only to procreation.

If at any stage of your life your religious beliefs seem in conflict with your sexuality, I'd recommend talking to someone like a Relate psychosexual counsellor who may be able to help you negotiate a satisfactory pathway through both.

In praise of mum and dad

Perhaps this section shouldn't close without a few words in praise of the role of mum and dad. One of the joys of a successful long-term relationship is that it fulfils a need that both of you have to be taken care of. Sometimes, at the end of a hard day, there is nothing more reassuring than your partner slipping into the role of a good 'parent' and listening patiently to your woes, reminding you that you are loved and doling out some grade A nurturing. It is only when one or both of you find yourself permanently stuck in the role of parent that your sex life is seriously at risk. As long as 'parent' is just one of the roles that you play in the relationship, your sex life will have every chance to flourish.

Being a couple without children

Increasingly, children are no longer an integral part of the deal in long-term relationships. Some couples are childless by choice, and the fact that women now have control over their fertility means that for the first time in generations women can safely choose not to have children. If you don't have children, it's likely that you will escape many of the pitfalls parents encounter in their sex lives, but that isn't to say that everything will be rosy.

If childlessness is not a choice, the struggle to have a child can decimate a previously happy sex life. Although 60 per cent of couples conceive within six months, the rest can take longer, and 15 per cent try for more than a year before conceiving. Infertility is categorised as the failure to conceive after a year of unprotected intercourse, and millions fall into this category.

Preparing yourself for parenthood is a big step, and when month after month you feel as though you have 'failed', it is not surprising that such a pressure can rapidly take its toll on your relationship and your sex life. As soon as you begin medical interventions to help you have a child, sex and pleasure can split apart abruptly as your bodies are scrutinised for flaws and then subjected, if you are a woman, to a high level of drugs and medical procedures.

How medical intervention can affect you

This can make you question the very roots of your masculinity and femininity, and all the assumptions you may have had about each other and yourselves can fall apart. If you do go on to have a baby, it will take time before you reassemble your relationship, and, as ever, it is vital to keep talking to each other, even when you really don't feel like it. This is for the simple reason that when communication between a couple stops flowing, trouble begins to brew. And issues that are not dealt with around this time will eventually resurface in the relationship, potentially made more dangerous by large dashes of anger and resentment accumulated as time goes on.

If you possibly can, try to have sex for fun or comfort outside the prescribed times when you are meant to be 'doing it' in order to assist conception. If this feels like a tall order, make sure that you continue to touch each other affectionately and carry on cuddling. Being stroked and cuddled will mean that you'll continue to release hormones that help you bond with each other. It will also reduce your stress levels and remind you of your feelings for each other, which may have become too focused on the intangible presence of the unborn child you both hope for.

It may take time to restart an enjoyable sex life after you have tried unsuccessfully to have a baby, and it is natural for your desire levels to dip, but if you continue to talk to each other about your feelings and worries, slowly your sexual feelings should return. If they don't, it may mean that there are underlying issues in the relationship, like anger or blame, for example, that need to be resolved.

If you remain childless it does not mean the end of your relationship. It does mean that you will have to make changes, though. Couples can invest years in trying for a baby, and the decision to stop can be intensely painful. The sense of loss and grief that stem from accepting that you won't have children may be overwhelming, or you may sense it as more of a continual dull ache.

Possess the loss; don't be possessed by it

Learning to be able to possess the loss, rather than being possessed by it, is a process that may take you months or years. Being able to accept that you cannot have a child who is genetically yours is a huge challenge for men and women. But couples that are able to do this successfully still play the role of 'caring parent' towards each other when it feels appropriate. Equally, they rarely shut down on all other relationships with children. Often they direct their energy into nieces and nephews or godchildren and ensure that they still play an important part in the lives of the next generation.

Reconnect your love

Restarting and enjoying sex after becoming parents can be difficult. As Val has shown, the psychological and practical barriers can prevent you feeling close. You may feel a sense of grief for the couple you were before your family came along, even though you want your baby very much. Or, if you are a woman and have had some problems in dealing with the physical effects of the birth – such as stitches, vaginal tears or breastfeeding difficulties – sex will be the last thing on your mind.

Once you are parents, you also have to manage your intimate life as the kids grow up. This is not easy, but if you go through stressful periods with your children (and who doesn't!), shared loving sex can help you to feel closer to your partner and relieve stressful feelings. Orgasm produces a natural relaxant that helps to defeat stress and anxiety, and regular touching promotes the release of oxytocin, a brain chemical that promotes bonding in couples.

Read the following case study and then take a look at some of the practical ideas that follow to help you maintain your sexual connection as you move from partners to parents.

CASE STUDY ·

Mel and Fred

Mel, 38, and Fred, 39, are the parents of three-year-old twins. They met when they were almost 30, and married a year later. They decided almost immediately to start trying for a family but were very disappointed when their longed-for baby did not appear. After ten months of trying for a baby, they approached their GP and were referred to the local fertility clinic. No underlying reason was found for their lack of a pregnancy, but Mel felt reassured by the investigations. She became pregnant within the next three months and, at her second scan, discovered she was having twins. She was amazed, although there are twins in Fred's family. Fortunately, the birth of the twins was straightforward and they were soon at home as a new family. But Mel was unprepared for the tiredness that followed the birth. She felt her whole day was spent changing and feeding her baby daughters. Fred returned to work after three weeks at home, leaving Mel to cope. Her mother was supportive, but Mel fell into bed at night exhausted by the day's tasks. Fred also felt tired. He had agreed to undertake overtime to give his new family some much needed extra cash, but often returned late in the evening.

For the first six months, Mel and Fred hardly thought about sex. They did make love a couple of times when the twins were about four months old, but it felt more like 'we ought to do this' than a real desire to do it. Mel was still breastfeeding and was disconcerted to discover that when she became aroused her breasts leaked milk. She felt confused about her sexual desires and Fred had trouble feeling close to Mel. As the twins grew older, Mel and Fred made love very infrequently. Mel tried to avoid thinking about the issue. When she did, she told herself it would work out when the kids were older. Fred was feeling resentful about the lack of sex but guilty that he felt this way. He could see how busy Mel was and felt bad about asking for love-making. Besides, he had to admit he was frequently very tired. They also spent most of their time talking about the children, with nearly every suppertime spent trying to work out what needed doing the next day. For two years, they rarely had an evening to themselves, and sex slid to the bottom of their priority list.

Now that the children are three years old, Mel and Fred feel depressed about the lack of a shared sex life. Talking about it has become very difficult, with Mel upset if Fred asks for sex and Fred worried that his level of desire for Mel is beginning to decline. They know they love each other, but cannot seem to find a way back to a joyful and satisfying intimate life. Mel wants to make love, but on the occasions she wants to she holds back from suggesting love-making to Fred. This is because she fears she could hurt his feelings as she has rejected him in the past. Therefore, neither initiates love-making. They feel stuck in a catch-22 situation – they would like sex but fear the repercussions of asking or refusing.

If, like Mel and Fred, you feel caught in the parent trap, all is not lost. Here is how to restore or reinvigorate your sexual relationship as you move from partners to parents.

The new parents

You may wonder when the new baby arrives whether you will ever have a sex life at all! The paraphernalia of bottles and nappies, broken nights and physical problems for the woman can completely stop sexual contact. However, there are some things you can do:

● If you are a woman, make sure you attend your postnatal check. This usually takes place six weeks after birth. If you are experiencing any vaginal soreness or discomfort in the pelvic area, tell the nurse or doctor. You should not attempt intercourse until you have the OK from this check. Getting a clean bill of health will help to restore your confidence and ease you back into thinking about love-making, albeit some time in the future.

- During the early days and weeks after the birth of your baby, sex will hardly be the first thing on your mind. Some people do feel sexy, and this could be related to the hormonal changes in the body, but most people feel tired and concentrated on their new child. However, this is the very time when you need to prepare for restarting your intimate life together. Weave lots of affection into your life together. Give your partner a kiss, cuddle up on the sofa and tell them how much you love them every day. Hold hands and talk about your relationship. This will help you to feel close to one another so that when you begin to think about love-making it will follow naturally.

- You may not be ready for intercourse but you could enjoy sensual touching and caressing. Offer to massage your partner and ask for the same for yourself. Stroke yourself in the bath or shower so you get used to the feel of soft caresses. Put some time aside to enjoy kissing and embracing in bed. Little and often is best at this time so find 30 minutes in your day when you can do this.

- When you feel ready for intercourse, use a good quality lubricant. Most chemists supply these and you can purchase 'natural feel' lubricant from the Internet at www.emotional bliss.co.uk.

- Talk to your partner about how you are feeling about sex. It is easy to forget to communicate on sex with everything else you have to think about. Try saying, 'I miss making love but I'm so tired at the moment that I don't think it would work out' or 'I really want a cuddle/massage/intimate touching but I'm not quite ready for intercourse.' Let them tell you how they are feeling. Avoid making a critical remark or saying, 'You are so insensitive to even be thinking about sex.' Even though love-making may not be immediately possible, it is crucial to say you fancy one another and want to make love. Just be careful that this is not too pressurising for your partner, but encouraging and loving.

Toddlers to school-age children

Once you have managed to resume love-making after the birth of a baby you may hope you have got it cracked! But toddlers can present a real challenge to your love life. A small baby cannot get out of its cot and burst in during your moment of passion, but a two-year-old can! Most parents can tell a tale of suddenly realising they have a visitor when they are 'in the act'. This can be a real passion killer, even if you can settle the child back to bed quickly. Here are a few ideas to help you survive this phase:

- Always use a bedtime routine so your child gets the idea that bed is for sleep. Bathe the children and read them a soothing story (keep exciting adventure stories for other times). Turn off the TV and avoid having one in their bedrooms. If you have two children sharing, put the younger child to bed first so they have a chance to nod off before the elder child joins them. Kiss them good night and gently, but firmly, tell them you will see them in the morning. Don't reward them with drinks or sweets if they get up in the evening. Just take them back to bed. If you can get a routine going, they will sleep longer and you will have a better chance of sharing some quality evening time as a couple.

- Make use of trusted friends and relatives as babysitters so you can have at least one evening a week to go out. A walk together is a good start, but you could work up to a drink in a quiet pub, a cinema visit or favourite meal out as you gain in confidence. This will keep your sense of intimacy alive, paving the way to successful sex when you feel ready.

● As Val mentions on page 81, consider fitting a lock to your bedroom door. You may not necessarily want to make love, but knowing your children cannot get in when they choose, only when you choose, allows you to feel close and less worried about being disturbed. Of course, you will need to take safety issues into account and use the lock sparingly (at those times when you might be interrupted, such as late evening) but careful use can allow you to feel psychologically prepared to understand you have a right to 'just us' time rather than being on tap 24 hours a day for your kids.

● As your child gets older it is likely that you will think about going back to, or starting, work. The complications of balancing home and work life can mean you put sex to the back of your mind. It can get lost in the tasks you have to do in the evenings, while weekends can be spent in a whirl of shopping, cleaning and cooking. During this phase, it is crucial that you think about your intimate life together. If sex drops to the bottom of the list it is no wonder that you will eventually feel dissatisfied with your love-making. Make dates in your diary to be together. These must be as important as anything else you do. You may not always make love during these dates, but you could enjoy cuddling and caressing one another. Without these precious times, you could find your sex life becomes another chore rather than a support to your life together.

School-age children

This category breaks down into two areas – pre-teens and teen-agers. Pre-teens will have a different set of issues to teenagers and they will affect you differently:

Pre-teens

● Pre-teens can take up a lot of time. Club membership (Scouts, dance classes or sports, for example) and visits to friends may mean you are an unpaid taxi service in the evenings. If you want relaxed space for the two of you, you need to limit the amount of time you spend driving your kids around in the evenings. Let them know you cannot do this non-stop. It could be helpful to set a limit on the amount of things they can belong to.

● If your children are at a friend's for a 'sleep-over' you can use the time to enjoy love-making without fear of disturbance. Set the scene with a favourite meal (but avoid heavy curries or traditional roasts as they will make you sleepy – the opposite of what you want!) and then take some time to get ready for love-making. Consider showering together or spending longer than usual in stroking and arousing each other. Pick a time when you feel sexiest – for example, you may feel more interested in sex first thing in the morning than in the evening. Serve your partner a sensual breakfast with fruit such as melon or figs, fruit juice (or Buck's fizz – orange juice and cham-pagne – if you are feeling extravagant) and soft-textured bread and warm butter to arouse their senses before sex.

● Be affectionate in front of your children. If you try to 'box' up your intimate life as separate from your children you may find it hard to be sexual when they are in the house at all – even if they are soundly asleep. Obviously, I'm not advocating full-on sex in front of the family, but a cuddle on the sofa or holding hands while you are out together signals to the kids that you have a private life and maintains the important idea that your closeness can exist alongside being parents.

Teenagers

The presence of teenagers in the family can produce two distinct effects. Most teenagers are 'grossed out' by the idea that their parents have sex. This can lead to you finding sex difficult if they are likely to hear you. Or you may find yourself longing for their carefree attitude to life, causing you to want to break out of sex that feels routine or boring.

● If you worry that your teenagers will hear you, or know you are making love, you need to think of strategies to allow you to enjoy sex without feeling constricted by their presence. For example, you might seize times to make love when you would not normally think of doing so. Choose a Saturday afternoon when they are shopping with friends, or a weekday evening when they are at a school event. You will need to be creative and to be ready to make love when you can. This can add to the excitement of love-making, giving it a 'naughty but nice' kick.

● If your teens' burgeoning sexuality causes you to feel rather lacklustre in bed, think of new ways to enliven your sex life together. Make love in different rooms and wear silky underwear. Use all your senses to arouse your partner – touch, scent and sight. Caress their whole body (rather than just the erogenous zones) and offer to experiment by reading sexy books together. Try Black Lace publications or *In the Buff* magazine, available from bookshops (and www.emotional bliss.co.uk). Don't force yourself to do anything you are not comfortable with to prove you are still sexy – just look for and enjoy some new ways of expressing yourself sexually.

- If your teenagers are 16 and over, now is the ideal time to have the odd weekend away. You may want to get a friend or neighbour to check that the children are OK while you are away, but a day or two in a B&B or self-catering cottage could boost your sense of togetherness and give you the freedom you need to explore new ways of making love. If this seems too expensive, do a deal with a friend who also has teenage children: explain you desperately need some quality time together (they are bound to be sympathetic) and ask if your teens can stay with them for the weekend. In return, you can do the same for them later. Don't be tempted to use your precious couple of days together choosing a new sofa or watching all the taped programmes you never see because the kids monopolise the TV. Get in lots of easy-to-eat foods, buy some exotic bath products and have a completely hedonistic weekend. Stay in bed the whole time if you want to, cuddle, kiss, and make love as much as feels natural.

It is crucial for you to maintain a healthy intimate life once you become a parent. If you concentrate so heavily on the children that your couple relationship feels second class, or feel swamped by the demands of work and family, it is easy to think 'My partner is an adult. They can look after him or herself. Sex will just have to wait and they will have to understand', you are treating sex as if it is another demand or drain on your resources. If this is how you feel, it is likely that your sex life has become a victim of your lack of care and attention. The truth is that if you have a loving intimate life it will sustain you through tough times. The affection of your partner when you have had a bad day at work, or gentle love-making that helps you realise there is more to life than worrying about whether the baby spits out his or her dinner, can make a huge difference to how content you feel in your relationship. Let your shared sexuality nurture your relationship and it will pay dividends on your sense of connection and love.

Case Study catch up

Mel and Fred found that they resolved many of their issues by adopting a diary approach to sex. They decided to put dates in their diary for spending time together, and to use this time (when they wanted) to make love. They also asked their mum to babysit more often so that they could have evenings together without interruption.

Your guide to sexual positions

If you are struggling with balancing work, family and leisure (if there is time for any!) sex can become very formulaic. Tiredness can cause you to do the same things every time you make love, causing love-making to feel routine and miles away from the exciting sex you may have had when you first started making love together. Alongside sensuous caressing and stroking, trying out different sexual positions can help you to feel like sexual, adult partners and not only parents going through the motions. If you are new parents, using a variety of sexual positions can also help you both discover the one most comfortable to accommodate sore breasts during breastfeeding and ensure you avoid exacerbating any residual vaginal soreness after childbirth, although you should always wait until any tears or cuts have healed before commencing intercourse again. Here is a selection of the most common sexual positions:

Man on top – 'missionary position'

With the woman beneath and the man on top, the missionary position is so called because it was the only position that missionaries told their converts was appropriate for intercourse! This position allows for full body contact and can feel very loving. Lots of couples revert to it at the end of love-making after using other positions for stimulation. The woman can vary vaginal sensation by widening or narrowing her legs, while the man can either lift himself up on his arms or lie flat against the woman's body.

It is less good for clitoral stimulation, as neither partner can easily reach the clitoris. Although it is possible for the man to slide in a finger or two to rub the clitoris as he penetrates his partner, it can be uncomfortable and difficult to achieve. It is easier for the woman to rub her clitoris in this position and can work well if the man lifts his body off his partner slightly.

Pelvic tilt or lift

In the pelvic tilt or lift position the man is on top and the woman places a pillow beneath her bottom. This position allows for controlled penetration, while allowing the vagina to be at the prime angle for the penis to enter. It can help if the man kneels or positions himself slightly below the vaginal entrance. One bed pillow gives a slight angle; two or more give a steeper incline to the vagina. Experiment with the number of pillows you find comfortable and arousing. A cylinder-shaped pillow is also good, as it tilts the pelvis and allows the woman to move around more. Place this shaped pillow just under the bottom, at the top of the thighs or in the small of the back. In this position, the man can slide his penis in slowly or fast according to his and his partner's pleasure. The woman can also hold the penis and guide it into the vaginal opening, controlling the speed the penis enters her at – ideal if you are recommencing intercourse after childbirth. This is also an excellent position for oral sex as the tilted pelvis allows the man unhindered access to the clitoris and labia. (For more on giving and receiving oral sex, see Your guide to oral sex in Chapter 7, Fear and Anxiety).

'The spoons'

The position known as the spoons is when both partners lie on their sides, with the man behind the woman. This position is good for warm and intimate love-making as the man can hold the full length of his body against the woman's back while embracing her with his arm wrapped around her breasts or hips. The woman should lie on her side, curling her legs slightly towards her chest. The man should form the same shape behind her, adjusting his penis so that he can enter the woman's vagina from the rear. The beauty of this position is that he can stimulate her clitoris with his fingertips by draping his arm over her hips. The woman can alter the angle at which the man enters the vagina by leaning forwards or backwards, or by arching her back a little. She can also open her legs or hold them closer together to vary the sensation for him and her.

In this position, couples can also achieve the elusive 'simultaneous orgasm' that people often feel is important to love-making, although this is not strictly necessary for mutually satisfying sex. The man can also whisper loving words in his partner's ear or kiss and nuzzle the back of her neck – very arousing for most women.

Woman on top, man beneath

There are a variety of these positions, so choose any that sound arousing. The one that most people think of is the woman sitting astride the man while he lies on his back. You do need to be flexible for this position, so if you have trouble with your knees or hip joints, avoid using it. If you are able, try squatting over your partner's erect penis and gradually lowering yourself on to it. If you can do this slowly, it feels incredibly erotic and sensual. Use plenty of lubricant and experiment with fast or slow vaginal entry. Squeeze the muscles at the entrance to the vagina when your partner is inside you. (This feels like trying to stop yourself going to the loo – practise it when you make love and your partner will enjoy the change in sensation. Some women feel it also improves orgasm. For more on this technique, see How to practise Kegel exercises, in Chapter 2, Self-esteem). You can also try lying down with your whole body covering your partner. Do this with legs spread wide apart or closed tightly together for different effects. Lift your bottom up and down fast or slow so that the penis moves in and out of the vagina, brushing over the entrance to the vagina. This area is rich with nerve endings (called the 'orgasmic platform' by therapists) and one of the key zones for stimulation, helping orgasm to occur. If you feel confident, try sitting on your partner with your back to him. The angle of the vagina means that this will feel very different from a face-to-face position, but can be highly arousing. Lean forward a little to increase pressure on the clitoral area.

Lying on side, face to face

This is a very intimate and relaxing position. It is easy to kiss and talk to one another, but less easy to stimulate the clitoris. The man can enter the vagina from the front while the woman lifts her upper leg over his hip. If she wishes, she can wrap her legs around him, but the lower leg can develop pins and needles if you stay in this position for a while! The man or woman can lean backwards to change the stimulation of the penis in the vagina, or you can use the position to slow things down before moving on to more vigorous activity.

How to be a sexy mum or dad

- *Don't live through your children.* Have your own life that gives you satisfaction. Your children will have their own choices and ideas to follow. You can love them without wanting to have a life through them.

- *Fence a bit of your life off from the kids.* Even if it is only a couple of hours in the evening or a weekend afternoon, creating this bit of space for the two of you will help you to feel you have a relationship that is about just the two of you rather than the family.

● Talk about what brought you together and remind yourselves of good intimate moments in the past. For example, say, 'Do you remember when we made love in the woods and were nearly caught?' or 'It was great when you wore that wonderful dress with the plunge neckline. It really turned me on.' This will connect you to your sexuality before children.

● Vary ways of being intimate. With time at a premium, try cuddling and kissing, touching intimately to arouse or to orgasm, making love speedily or slowly when you have more time. Boost your daily affection towards one another.

● Compliment your partner on their body. If you are a man and your partner's body has changed since childbirth, let her know you still find her attractive and desirable. Tell her that you like her breasts and hips. If you are a woman, return the compliments so that your partner knows he is still attractive to you.

● Go on dates together. A drink at the local, a cinema visit or a meal out will help you feel closer to one another. Take advantage of offers of babysitting from friends and family you trust. Wear the kind of clothes you feel attractive in and that are different from those you wear during the day.

● Use massage oils and lubricants to help you enjoy sex. Awaken your senses with perfume or creams so that you don't feel immersed in baby sick or adolescent smelly socks!

KEY MESSAGE

It can take time for parents to feel sexy again after childbirth. Give yourself time, put your relationship first and hang on to what brought you together. Your family depends on the strength of your relationship. Emotional and sexual investment in your partnership is effort well spent towards the security of your family.

CHAPTER 4

stress

. . . .

Stress is one of the major reasons couples give for abandoning their sex lives. 'I'm too stressed out to have sex,' one partner, or even both, might say, climbing into bed at the end of a tiring day. 'I can't even think about sex.' Sometimes the message is unspoken. But flinching or turning your back on your partner when they reach out for a sexual touch also speaks volumes.

Of course, if your sex life has dwindled into a repetitive pattern that has stopped bringing one or both partners much pleasure or comfort, it is an attitude that makes perfect sense. Why would anyone want to add another activity to a life that is already bursting at the seams, especially if that activity feels like yet another chore?

Tackle sex-life stress on two fronts

The key to handling the problem of stress affecting your sex life is to tackle it on two fronts. The first is to begin to get a grip on your stress levels in your work and family life; the second is to establish a different pattern of love-making with your partner, so that sex becomes something that relieves stress instead of creating it.

Stress accounts for 6.5 million lost working days in the UK and doubtless many more millions of passion-free nights. Stress means different things to different people and we vary hugely in our ability to cope with it. But whatever it is that triggers your stress, it will probably make you feel that you aren't coping effectively with the difficulties in front of you. As a result you may find yourself overwhelmed by a sense of crisis, and as though you are stretched way beyond your normal limits. And as most of us know, it is not a good feeling.

Stress is not an evil baddy

But before we start to portray stress as the evil baddy on a mission to wipe out our sex lives, it is important to remember that a certain amount of stress can be extremely useful. It can act as a motivator to get us going and drive us to achieve goals at home and work. In fact, stress has its origins in nature's desire to equip us to survive in a hostile environment.

What we feel as stress waiting for a delayed commuter train, for example, is our in-built 'fight or flight' syndrome, designed to enable us to battle with or run away from predators. Understandably, kicking your heels in your business suit at Waterloo station for the late-running 6.15 p.m. to Guild-ford feels light years away from being confronted by a hungry sabre-toothed tiger. But our physiological response is the same. Your body is ready to act because you face a real, imag-ined or suspected threat. Your cardiovascular and respiratory systems, for example, are preparing you to pick up the near-est club and whack your attacker, or for you to run as fast as you can in the opposite direction.

The physical changes

Among many physical changes stress produces, the following take place:

- Your adrenal glands secrete more adrenaline, cortisol and other hormones into your blood. This diverts your body's resources from your internal organs, such as your stom-ach, to your muscles.

- Your breathing becomes deeper and more rapid to increase oxygen supply to your muscles.

- Blood drains from your skin, which is why we go pale when we are scared.

- The nervous and hormonal actions trigger changes in bowel movements, which is why stress can cause nausea, diarrhoea and is often associated with irritable bowel syn-drome.

Short-term stress can be helpful

Some people, such as athletes and actors, use stress to boost their performance, and fear that without nervous tension before a game or a show they will become complacent and not give their best. They run their race or act their part, knowing that they are riding high on the physical boost their body has given them. So in this context, short-term stress can be enormously helpful.

But many of us have no immediate outlet for using up our physical responses triggered by our fight-or-flight reflex. This instinct doesn't distinguish between an attack by a bunch of Vikings on an awayday to pillage and burn our village, and a nagging, critical boss (or even a nagging, critical voice inside our own head). We can't easily thump the boss or run out of the office (or silence the voice), and as a result our fight-or-flight reflex remains active for long stretches of time. This drains our physical, emotional and mental reserves. And it is easy for us to end up exhausted.

So it's not surprising then, that as a result we are not in the mood for sex. Good sex is about giving, and if you feel that you are emotionally and physically bankrupt because you are so stressed, it is understandable that your desire for sex will decline or be eradicated totally.

Relationships between partners are also a source of stress and the chances are that if it is your relationship that is causing your fight-or-flight reflex to spark into action too often, sex will not be a priority on your agenda.

Stress and arguments

Interestingly, when a man and woman row, usually the man becomes more stressed by the argument than the woman. One study showed that when men and women were deliberately treated rudely and then told to relax for 20 minutes, male blood pressure surged and stayed elevated until the man was given a chance to retaliate. But women facing the same treatment were able to calm down during those 20 minutes.

When you consider that a row takes a greater physical toll on a man, it is understandable that men are more likely than women to attempt to avoid it. It also explains why women, who are better able to handle the stress, tend to be the ones to bring up sensitive issues.

So whether your stress comes from inside or outside your relationship, if it is having a negative impact on your sexual relationship with your partner, it is time to examine different ways of managing it better so that both of you benefit.

Outside your relationship

Let's look first at ways of reducing stress outside your relationship so that it does not begin to impinge on your feelings about yourself and your partner. Psychologists describe certain strategies of handling stress as 'assertive coping', which in layman's terms means that instead of feeling powerless and overwhelmed by the circumstances around you, you deliberately take steps to change or improve your situation.

There are three main processes behind this. You can:

● Change your environment

- Change your behaviour

- Change your response to the stress

Changing your environment

For some people this might mean 'down-shifting' and moving away from corporate city life to working from home in a country village. This can work wonderfully well, or it might mean exchanging one set of stresses – overcrowding, noise and pollution – for another set – isolation, too much quiet and the whiff of manure from the field opposite.

Changing your environment in small ways can be more successful. If you feel that your life is a mess, put aside a weekend to de-clutter your house, for example, and you may well find that more ordered surroundings help you function better. Of course, if you thrive on piles of books, newspapers and memorabilia, this won't work. But there will probably be at least one or two things you can shift around or clear, even if they are just dates in your diary, that will give you a little more breathing space.

Changing your behaviour

Poor time-management is a major cause of stress. Spending hours sorting a trivial problem is often a distraction from the real difficulties you might face, and contributes to make matters worse by diverting your attention from them. Time-management has been a buzzword in business life for years and there are plenty of books that offer techniques to improve the way you spend your time. Read at least a couple and be prepared to try some different styles before you find the one that works for you.

Bearing in mind that this book is about sex and not business, I'd include the following recommendations, too.

- Use one diary for work and home, rather than trying to juggle separate ones. And make sure you diarise time to spend with your partner. This could be a meal out, a trip to the cinema, or an evening in together when you ignore domestic chores in favour of sharing a bottle of wine and a DVD. Actually writing down this time together as you would a work appointment might not feel spontaneous or romantic, but our brains seem to pay better attention to written information, and you have a much greater chance of spending an enjoyable time together if you have planned for it in this way. If you don't believe me, just try it for a month and see the difference it makes.

- Keep a 'to do' list which includes things you can do for your partner as well as yourself. Keep your priorities up to date, which may mean taking a few moments to rewrite it every day. If you want to be super-efficient and stress-free, number each task from one to ten, say, and start each day with task number one. Then move to task two and so on. Anything left at the end of the day goes on the following day's list at number one. This may be a technique too far for some, but it does ensure that the jobs you don't fancy doing never get put off indefinitely.

- Learn to say 'no'. Saying 'yes' to everything and then getting stressed about it is not a route to making people like you. This applies to your sexual relationship as much as your interaction with work and friends. Think about it. Your 'yes' doesn't mean very much if you can't say 'no', does it? If the thought of saying 'no' to anything fills you with panic, try saying 'no' to small things at first, and instead of feeling guilty, give yourself a pat on the back for being true to yourself.

If you are saying 'no' to sex, explain your reasons tenderly to your partner, and if your 'no' is a response to a problem between you, put aside some time to discuss it properly.

Changing your response to stress

We all have to accept that stress will never go away, but we can learn to handle it so that it is no longer a major problem. A feeling of control is the crucial difference between people who believe they can tackle their problems and those who feel helpless. Psychologists explain the difference between people by noting whether the person has an internal or external 'locus of control'.

People with an internal locus of control believe that they achieve a given outcome, whether it is a satisfying relationship or a fulfilling life, through their own actions. People with an external locus of control believe the exact opposite – that outcomes depend mainly on luck or the actions of others.

So 'internal' people tend to feel in command of a situation, while 'externals' feel the situation controls them. It follows, then, that people with an internal locus of control are better able to adapt and cope with difficulties. In fact, one researcher reported that an internal locus of control partly protected holocaust survivors from depression, anxiety and other psychological problems. You have only to read the work of Primo Levi, and others who have written about their experiences in the Nazi concentration camps during the Second World War, to understand that you still have choices, even in the most dire circumstances, and believing this is one of the keys to psychological survival.

Ironically, acquiring this sense of being in charge of your life, rather than at the mercy of others, can be stressful in itself, simply because the process of change, no matter how beneficial, is stressful.

Tips to combat stress

If you are stressed by your sexual relationship, try these suggestions to improve the situation:

- *Limit the number of changes that you make*. Don't try to turn everything in your sex life upside down because at present you are feeling stressed. Not everything will be contributing to your stress. Indeed, it may be only one or two things that are at the route of your problem. Make one small change at a time. You may find that it sets in motion all sorts of other positive changes in its wake.

- *Don't expect immediate results*. You may be surprised by how quickly making one or two changes reduces your stress level, but be prepared to wait before the benefits kick in properly. 'Limit your expectations but not your effort' is the best motto to abide by.

- *Make only necessary changes*. When you are feeling stressed, you can think that you've got your whole life wrong, and as a result you may be tempted to alter some aspects of your life unnecessarily (like deciding to seek a new sexual partner or embarking on an affair). Pay attention to the areas that are bothering you most in your current relationship and see how the rest settles into place.

If you have gone off sex because you feel stressed by your partner, try the following listening exercise so that you can begin to establish between you what is going wrong:

> Agree to spend 15 minutes listening to your partner, taking it in turns, and while they speak, you just listen. This won't work if you are very angry, by the way: if your heart rate exceeds 100 beats a minute you won't be able to hear what your partner is saying, no matter how hard you try. Take a 20-minute break before you try to communicate again.

If you are feeling generally stressed, resist the urge to think that a holiday will put everything right. One poll found that 53 per cent of those questioned said that taking a holiday was for them the most stressful life event over the last year. Instead, consider trying some of the stress-management techniques outlined below. As ever, try several and use what works for you.

Meditation and relaxation

Practising meditation focuses the mind in a state of relaxed awareness. It is linked to spirituality, but you don't have to believe in God in order to receive its physiological and psychological benefits. In Europe, some insurance companies offer lower premiums to meditators, as scientists have proved that meditation lowers the blood pressure and boosts the immune system.

There are many different forms of meditation. Simply sitting still with your back straight, closing your eyes and following the progress of your breath is one approach. It's best if you can find a quiet room, where you won't be distracted by the phone, the TV, or other people.

Set aside anything between 15 and 30 minutes (15 minutes is usually enough if you are a beginner) and try to meditate at least once a day. If you can manage it twice, you'll probably experience the benefits sooner. You can learn a mantra meditation (where you repeat a word or sound inside your head) from a teacher, or you can choose your own word, such as 'love' or 'peace'.

Meditation is not the same as deep relaxation, although it is often mixed up with it. Relaxation induces a state of calmness, which is necessary to meditation, but meditation brings clarity of mind that is not always present when you are relaxing. The best sort of relaxation, though, is not dozing in front of the television, but doing something that brings you real pleasure, whether it is singing in a choir or baking a cake. (If it nurtures your creativity it will be an even more effective stress-beater.)

Massage

Whether your stress comes from outside your relationship, or whether you and your partner are finding things tough, if you can still like each other enough to share a massage, you will be benefiting your relationship on several levels.

The first point to make clear is that a massage need not be a direct route to sex (unless that is what both of you want). In fact, if you are trying to rekindle a sex life, simply touching each other to bring pleasure, without the perceived pressure of sex, is a wonderfully gentle reintroduction to the pleasure each other's bodies can bring.

When we touch each other, a hormone called oxytocin is released into the bloodstream, decreasing stress levels and increasing sex hormones. In women this raises sexual responsiveness and in men it boosts the sensitivity of their penis and improves their erection.

So don't confine a massage to a five-minute rub of the shoulders before getting on with the seemingly more important business of having sex. Quite apart from the fact that it is a fantastic stress-reliever, a massage can be an intensely sensual experience by itself. Buy some massage oil and take time to find out what your partner likes. Age is no barrier to enjoying massage; in fact if your joints are aching and your back isn't as strong as it used to be, a massage will be an even more worthwhile investment of your time.

If you have never given or received a massage before, it can be a good idea to start by giving your partner a hand and foot massage. This is often very pleasurable for the recipient, and it doesn't feel as daunting as an entire naked body when you aren't sure quite where to start. One more suggestion for stress-relieving massage: accompany your hand movements with a soundtrack of compliments. Praise any aspect of your partner's body that you like, from the curve of their shoulder to the dimple at the back of their knee. This level of intimacy distinguishes your massage from that of a professional masseur, and if you have been together for a while, it can act as a reminder to both of you that although your bodies may have become familiar over the years, they are still special and unique.

Music

An excellent stress-reliever, music has the capacity to slow your brainwaves and make you feel more calm and relaxed. Your skin becomes more sensitive to touch and temperature, and music played at a rate of about 60 beats a minute has the ability to lower heart rate, reducing breathing and brainwaves to the same level as during meditation, which is slightly slower than the average resting heart rate of 72 to 80 beats a minute. Pieces by Mozart, Tchaikovsky and Chopin, as well as light jazz and most New Age music generally play at 60 beats a minute or slower. Rock is much faster, causing your brain-waves to cycle faster and making you want to speed up whatever you are doing. Playing a selection of your favourite music when you are stressed will help lift your mood and enable you to relax. Don't underestimate the power of music to make you feel differently within a surprisingly short space of time.

Better sex without stress

As Val has suggested, the link between sex and stress is not simple. Some positive stress in our lives is crucial. Stress can be a motivator, pushing us to take occasional exciting risks or complete an arduous task. Without motivation, we would all spend our lives under the duvet, dreading the real world outside the door! It also helps us to enjoy sex. The pleasurable muscle tension and butterflies in the stomach as we become aroused are a form of stress, preparing us for sexual excitement and satisfaction.

However, problems occur when our lives are flooded with stress – either from an internal source (worry, for example) or external (taking an important exam, for example). This can prevent our normal response to sexual arousal. Chronically high levels of cortisol in the body, a stress-related hormone that is linked to our immune systems, is thought to depress sexual interest. So if you are always stressed, with little relaxation or sense of release in your life, your sexual desire levels can plummet.

CASE STUDY ·

Paul and April

Paul and April are both in their mid-forties with three children aged 15, 12 and ten. Paul is a salesperson for a pharmaceutical firm, driving thousands of miles a year, while April works as a teaching assistant in a college for children with learning disabilities. Some years ago, they bought a larger house, stretching their capacity to pay the mortgage to the limit. They now have debts on credit and shop cards. April would like to work part-time but they simply cannot afford for her to do this. Paul finds his work very demanding and he is frequently tired at the end of the week. On top of this, the two eldest children are flexing their teenage muscles, and April and Paul often have to cope with disagreements about what time the 15-year-old can come home and where the 12-year-old can go to hang out.

It is therefore no surprise that their sex life is lacking. They are tired, often feel that the other does not support them in managing the kids and worried and resentful about their financial situation. Finding the time for love-making, and then feeling in the right mood, is tough for both of them. They sometimes argue about sex, but more often weeks pass where they avoid raising the subject. They have reached a situation of stalemate where neither of them wants to talk about sex in case it makes things worse, but they also know that they do not want things to stay this way for ever.

Beat your stress demons

One of the reasons for stress taking a hold on your life is that it usually creates a vicious circle: you become stressed over an event or problem; you stew on it wondering what to do about it; this causes more stress, especially if you do not immediately know how to solve the difficulty, and soon you are caught in a cycle of stress. Breaking the vicious cycle is the only way to deal with the situation.

Here are ten stress-busting ideas to get you started. Although these are not obviously linked to sexual feelings, they will help to reduce your stress levels. Sex will then be more attractive to you.

1. *Do look for your personal stress triggers*. For example, Paul finds an especially long drive on a Friday evening, just when he most wants to get home, triggers feelings of anger and

irritation. Make a note of your triggers and think about how they might be changed. For example, you could talk to your boss about changing a pattern of work, arrange a special meal with your partner, or do something active to counteract the physical tension you may experience because of stress. (Physical exercise can also relax your mind, helping you to switch off from worry, at least for a while.)

2. *Do take notice of the messages your body is telling you*. If you are coping with stress, your body will let you know. You may have muscle aches, headaches that seem to grip your forehead and shoulders, experience stomach aches or irritable bowel syndrome and generally feel tired and exhausted. Dry eyes and skin can also be a symptom of stress, as can lack of lubrication during love-making. This happens because your immune system is undermined by stress. Muscles do not relax properly and your lymph system works below par. If you notice these kinds of symptoms on a regular basis, chances are that you are suffering from chronic stress. Take notice of what your body is feeling. Ignoring the warning signs can, over time, lead to a complete collapse.

3. *Do think positively*. One of the side effects of stress is that you experience a more negative way of thinking. For example, you may find yourself thinking 'How can my partner fancy me? I am tense and grumpy the whole time.' Change this way of thinking. Look at every situation from both sides – positive as well as negative. If you worry that your partner does not fancy you, think about the warmth and affection they show you. Tell them what they mean to you and invite them to let you know your importance in their life. Studies suggest that people who think positively are less likely to suffer from illness, live longer, and cope with setbacks more effectively.

4. ***Make space in your life to relax***. Most people think of relaxing as lying prone doing nothing. While this might be true for some people, relaxing can also be active. If you feel stressed out by work or family demands, allow space in your life to do something that nurtures you and has little value other than personal pleasure. You may take up pottery or gardening, snowboarding or jogging or join a film club. The trick is to find something that does not have deadlines or demands attached that you can lose yourself in. The reason that this is important is that these are the very attributes you also need to enjoy sex. Sex should not seem like a chore, or one where you are giving with little reward. If you can practise letting go by relaxing in other parts of your life, sex will also seem less pressured and difficult.

5. ***Do tell your partner what you are feeling***. Stress can make you feel as if you are a tight drum of anxiety, anger, or frustration, trying to contain every problem inside yourself. Your partner may see your stress but not understand why it is happening. It helps to unload your feelings and thoughts so your partner understands where you are coming from. Beware of expecting them to act as a dumping ground for your emotions, but sharing your tension can relieve feelings, leaving you freer to enjoy sex when you want to.

6. ***Do give yourself positive messages***. If you are stressed during love-making, you may find yourself thinking 'I wish this was over' or 'I'll never have an orgasm because I am too tired.' Instead of these negative thoughts, try 'His/her stroking feels wonderful', 'I really love being kissed' or 'I know I am tired but love-making makes me feel special and cared for.' It takes an effort of will to do this. If you have spent years filling your head with reasons to avoid sex, thinking differently takes practice. Every time you are aware of a negative image entering your head, think of a positive one to replace it. You could even try writing these down to remind you of why sex can be healing and relaxing.

7. ***Do try meditating together***. I am not suggesting you take up intense meditation because this can take years to accomplish. But you could find it helpful to put a little time aside to relax together. As Val has suggested, find a place to sit comfortably and gradually slow down your breathing. You might find it helpful to hold hands or put a hand on each other's chest as you breathe together. Use the count of three as you breathe in, hold the breath for three, and then breathe out to the count of three. Do this together for 15 minutes every day. Empty your head of worries, replacing them with a pleasant image, or think of a black velvet curtain passing across your mind. You may choose to make love after your meditation or simply use it to improve your sense of closeness to one another. You may feel a bit foolish at first as it is a new piece of behaviour, but regular practice will improve this experience. Many couples describe it as feeling like a special place they can go to together that is intensely private and important.

8. ***Do create your own space***. Stress often produces a feeling of invasion; that thoughts and feelings are filling your head but have nowhere to go. These feelings can be worse if you have nowhere in your home that feels like your space. This is particularly important for love-making. Take time to create the kind of bedroom (or other room you tend to make love in) that helps you to feel 'this reflects us'. Choose colours and fabrics that you know say something about the two of you. Be as individual as you like, but make sure the room is a place you can be in and feel relaxed. Keep the idea of love-making alive in

your special room by using sensuous textures for bedcovers and curtains, and pictures that have an erotic quality (arty nudes or provocative classic paintings such as *The Girl with the Pearl Earring* or any Renoir nude, for example). Avoid pictures of film or sport celebrities, harsh colours, or fluorescent lighting.

9. *Do allow sensuality to be a part of your life*. Have you ever wondered why pop videos and adverts often feature a well-aimed wind machine sweeping over a long-haired lovely or fluttering a diaphanous skirt? It's because we know that the breeze passing over our skin is caressing and mildly arousing. When we see these images in a film or photo, our unconscious responds to the sexual sensation of air passing over the skin, encouraging a positive response to the product or song the image conjures up. Stress can cause us to feel numb to the sensuous in the world around us. This can have a detrimental affect on our sex life because we 'shut down' our sexual antennae, preventing us from responding to our partner or our personal sense of sexuality. View every day as an opportunity to enjoy sensual pleasures. For example, relish the warm breeze on your arms and neck as you walk along the road. Eat slowly, allowing every taste bud to respond to the flavours of the food you have chosen. Wear clothes that feel good on the skin (soft fleece – often found in sweatshirts – silks, velvets, crisp cotton and warm wool, anything that gives your skin a thrill). Use a favourite scent or aftershave to stimulate you, especially if it is one you often wear for special occasions or that your partner likes. Be aware of pleasant scents around you, such as the aroma of flowers and favourite foods. Play music that gives you a sense of enjoyment in being alive – rock with a bass beat, intricate classical music or pop that

reminds you of happy times can all improve your sensual response. Lastly, enjoy what you see around you. Drink in favourite views, visit an art gallery, or read a book containing sexy scenes.

10. *Do reward yourself more often*. Chronic stress can often cause a loss of self-esteem. This can spill over into your sex life, causing you to feel you do not deserve pleasurable love-making. You can overcome this by allowing yourself small rewards during the day. If you complete a task, allow yourself five minutes' reflection time. Have a cup of tea or coffee, look out the window at the sky or garden and tell yourself, 'I did that well.' It doesn't matter if the task was simple (such as sorting the washing) or more complicated (such as completing a project at work), rewarding yourself for your effort with positive messages throughout the day really can help you see yourself as capable and satisfied. You can also do this during and after sex. While caressing, or being caressed, tell yourself, 'This is lovely.' After love-making, tell your partner how much you enjoyed it and tell yourself, 'I am a good lover and help my partner to feel good about him or herself.'

Some people use self-reward as a cover for low self-esteem. Every time the going gets tough, they go shopping! This rarely has the positive effect they hope for, as they feel guilty about the money they have spent or realise that a new pair of shoes will not mask the unhappiness within. Using personal affirmation in the way I have described above helps to counteract the ache within, making sex more interesting and fulfilling.

Common sexual problems

Stress can contribute to sexual problems. Many sexual difficulties are a mixture of physical, emotional and mental issues. But stress can make all sexual problems much worse. If you or your partner suffers from problems with (for men) maintaining an erection, premature ejaculation, delayed ejaculation, or (for women) a lack of orgasm or painful sex, here are some guidelines to help you take steps towards solving these problems:

Male sexual problems

Erection difficulties

Most men experience a loss of erection occasionally. A night of over-indulgence of alcohol, tiredness or a short-term worry can all lead to an 'off night' when an erection either fails to appear or disappears partway through love-making. If this happens to your partner, be sympathetic (never critical), reassure him and put it down to experience. (Sometimes waiting an hour or so before making love will put things right, especially if alcohol is the chief cause of the problem.) However, if you or your partner has recurring problems with a loss of erection that last for more than three months, you need to take action. The first thing to do is to make an appointment to see your GP. This is because a gradual loss of erection that comes on slowly over a period of time can be an indicator of a more serious health problem. For example, diabetes and multiple sclerosis both often lead to a loss of erection, as do problems with the circulatory system. Explain exactly what is happening to your GP and ask for a general health check. Although your GP will know what prescription drugs you are taking, always tell him or her what non-prescription drugs you are using as well as complementary medicines. Some drugs, such as beta-blockers, can cause a temporary loss of erection. Your GP may be able to give you a type of your prescription drug that is less likely to interfere with your sexual performance.

If your health check does not show up any medical reasons for your loss of erection, and you lost your erection fairly quickly (suddenly and unexpectedly on more than a couple of occasions), and you can still get reliable erections during masturbation or on waking, your erection loss is more likely to be psychological in origin. You need to relax more and avoid all pressure to perform sexually. Ask you partner for lots of massage and love play so that you have time to enjoy the run up to intercourse. Try not to focus on the act of penetration. Instead, caress and stimulate each other with hands and lips for as long as you wish. It can help to agree not to have intercourse for a couple of weeks (but stick to this time limit). Instead, practise mutual masturbation to orgasm or pretend you are back in the early days of your relationship and enjoy extended petting sessions, over and under clothes. This will help you to get over the fear of failing your partner, often called 'performance pressure' by sex therapists, and restore your confidence in your erection.

If this simple plan does not do the trick, try the 'wax/wane' method:

> Put aside three separate hours during a week for intimate time with your partner. Enjoy touching and caressing each other until you have an erection (even a soft one will do). Lie on your back and ask your partner (using a lubricant) to rub your penis until you are fully or almost erect. Then ask her to stop. Let the erection subside a little, and ask her to do the same again.
>
> Do this two or three times, letting the erection subside a little each time. On the last time, ask her to masturbate you to ejaculation.

This method 're-educates' you into realising that even a lost erection can return. (You can also follow this programme through masturbation. Try after a relaxing bath and when you are certain of peace and quiet. The only drawback is that you might still lose the erection with a partner if, for some reason, you start to worry that you are not getting things right.) Once your confidence is improved, try the same technique during penetration. Enter your partner when you are hard, rest until your penis becomes soft, thrust until you get hard and repeat two or three times, ejaculating when you wish. This technique takes a little time to learn, and you should continue with your programme for at least a month.

Restoring an erection through this programme can be extremely successful, but if you find it still does not work, consider seeing a psychosexual therapist. Contact one via the British Association for Sexual and Relationship Therapists (www.basrt.org.uk) or Relate (Yellow Pages under 'Counselling/ Advice' or www.relate.org.uk).

A word about Viagra: Viagra has become the treatment synonymous with erection problems. At the first sign of erection problems, many men race to their GP to get these little blue pills. There is no doubt that Viagra has changed and enhanced the life of thousands of men across the globe, many of whom thought that they might never have an erection again. For them, and their partners, Viagra has been a wonder drug. But it doesn't suit everyone and some men have found that integrating it into a loving relationship has proved troublesome. The difficulty is that although getting an erection is a pre-requisite of intercourse, the whole act of making love is more complicated than just having a reliable erection. For example, Barry and Florence had been married for 26 years when Barry saw his doctor about losing his erection. His GP prescribed Viagra, which allowed Barry to get a reliable erection for the first time in three years. He was delighted, but Florence's reaction was less favourable. She had become used to Barry's erection difficulties, and privately thought their sex life had improved because Barry was more willing to caress her to orgasm when he could not penetrate her. Now he had his erection back, he seemed to want to give up the touching and stroking and just penetrate her instead. Florence began to avoid sex, causing Barry to feel angry and disappointed. He could not understand her response, and they began to argue about sex. Eventually, Florence booked a joint appointment with a psychosexual therapist who helped them to integrate Viagra into their sex life.

If you encounter this problem when using Viagra, make sure that you spend lots of time caressing and cuddling before attempting intercourse. Only use the Viagra when you both have time to enjoy its effects. Take time to talk about how it might alter your sexual pattern and behaviour. This is especially important if you or your partner has not had an erection for some time and you have either abandoned sex or, like Florence and Barry, adapted what you do together to take account of the erection loss. Viagra can be a fantastic boon, but it is worth thinking through how it will affect your sexual relationship in the long term.

Premature ejaculation

PE, or premature ejaculation is extremely common, particularly in the early stages of a new sexual relationship. Young men are more likely to suffer from it than older men are, but it can be a problem that lasts for years. It used to be thought that it was chiefly caused by an over-eagerness to reach orgasm, but new theories suggest that this may not be the full story. Recent advances in drug treatments for depression have shown that some drugs prescribed to alleviate depression also help to prevent premature ejaculation. If you have problems with PE it could help to visit your GP for a course of these new drugs, but taking any drug is not problem-free and many antidepressants also cause a loss of interest in sex. Talk to your health professional so that you can weigh up the pros and cons. As with erection problems, a check-up could rule out any medical problems that could be contributing to your premature ejaculation.

If there is no obvious medical issue, stress and tiredness can lead to PE, as you are less likely to be in control when you are exhausted. In the main though, the chief cause is anxiety. The more you worry it is going to happen, the more likely it is to occur. Forget the old wives' tales that tell you to think about work, or count backwards to diminish arousal and 'last longer'. These techniques only turn off your engagement with the act of love-making and can cause a feeling of dissociation that is upsetting for you and your partner. Instead, try the 'stop/start' technique. This has similarities to the 'wax/wane' technique for erection problems, but has a different result. This technique will help you to recognise the 'moment of inevitability' – that is when you are about to ejaculate. (Interestingly, the moment of orgasm for a man precedes actual ejaculation by less than a second.) Once you know this, you can stop when you want to and extend love-making to suit both of you.

Spend some time caressing and stimulating each other so that you feel turned on and sexually excited. Lie on your back and ask your partner to rub and caress your penis with her hand (use a lubricant). Do this until you start to feel that you might be about to 'come'. When you experience this sensation, tell her to stop arousal immediately. You can also use a signal (such as tapping the bed), if you prefer. Let the desire to ejaculate recede, and then do the same thing again. Do this three times and then ejaculate.

When you start this practice you may have 'accidents' – that is, you ejaculate during the 'stop/start'. Don't worry about this. Just keep practising until you are able to recognise the feelings that lead up to your orgasm, and stop. You will need to carry out this technique three times a week for at least a month. You can do it through masturbation, but you may find the problem re-emerges during love-making. Once you have mastered the technique through hand stimulation, try it during penetration. Do the same thing – stopping and starting while in the vagina. Gradually, you will feel more confident and in control of your orgasm. You will need the support and help of your partner, so explain why you want to do this and how beneficial it could be for her. If you feel you need extra support, contact the British Association for Sexual and Relationship Therapists (www.basrt.org.uk) or Relate (Yellow Pages under 'Counselling/Advice' or www.relate.org.uk).

Delayed or slow ejaculation

This male sexual problem is less common than erection problems or premature ejaculation, but, statistically, it seems to be increasing. Anxiety about the security of the relationship can cause this effect or problems in relating to women because of unresolved issues from the past. It is also important that you have a thorough check-up by your GP, as some delayed ejaculation can be caused by medical conditions or the side effects of prescription and non-prescription drugs. (Strong painkillers can deaden sexual response, leading to this problem.) Most men with this difficulty have no problem in achieving an erection and can thrust in the vagina for ages, but do not ejaculate. Some men with delayed ejaculation can ejaculate only after intercourse when alone. This might sound like a bonus for a woman as she can enjoy lengthy sex, but in practice, many women find they get sore through extended friction in the vagina or feel they have somehow let their partner down because he is not able to ejaculate. If you are a woman who experiences this, you may also feel let down that your partner has to masturbate in order to ejaculate.

Of the male sexual problems, and where there is no underlying medical problem, psychosexual therapy is the treatment of choice. Delayed ejaculation can be resistant to couple-alone interventions. Therapy can help because the man probably needs to explore his anxiety about penetration and ejaculation (sometimes related to fear of impregnating the woman or guilt about sex) to resolve the issue. The man can try masturbating with his partner in the room, or ask her to masturbate him, so that he gets used to the idea that it is OK to ejaculate in her presence, but therapy will help deal with these issues. Contact the British Association for Sexual and Relationship Therapists (www.basrt.org.uk) or Relate (Yellow Pages under 'Counselling/ Advice' or www.relate.org.uk).

Female sexual problems

Difficulty in reaching orgasm

It's not unusual for a woman to find it difficult to achieve orgasm through masturbation and/or during love-making and penetration. As many as 20 per cent of the women who attend sex therapy either have never had an orgasm or find it difficult to achieve orgasm with their partner or during masturbation. Some problems with reaching orgasm are linked to a lack of trust in a partner, stress that prevents a woman from relaxing, or problems in a relationship that cause sex to feel unsatisfying. For example, if you argue about money, or how to manage the children, you may find it hard to enjoy sex with a partner with whom you feel angry. Sorting out these problems could help you to achieve an orgasm with your partner.

If you find it difficult to reach orgasm on a regular basis, here are some tips to help you. However, they will work only if your relationship is secure and you feel stress-free. (Always use a lubricant during masturbation or love play with a partner.)

Practise touching your labia and clitoris in the bath. Use the natural lubrication of the water to help you rub and stroke this highly sensitive area. Take your time. Lay back, close your eyes, and let the sensations wash over you. (Avoid using bubble bath or soap as this can cause vaginal soreness.) You can also try this in the shower. Position the jet of water directly on the clitoral area for arousal and stimulation.

During masturbation, try tensing and relaxing the muscles in your legs as you become aroused. This can improve sensation and mimics what happens naturally during orgasm. The muscle tension can help you to feel more sexually excited and is especially effective in the vulval area. Try tensing and relaxing the muscles at the entrance to the vagina in fast succession. You should notice a sense of warmth and gentle arousal.

When making love, place a pillow under your bottom. This allows full access to the vulva and clitoris for you and your partner. As he caresses you, place your hand on his hand showing him how firmly or softly you like to be caressed.

Ask your partner to sit up in bed (or on the floor) with his legs apart. Position yourself with your back to him, sitting between his legs. Lay back so that your back is against his chest. Now ask him to stimulate your clitoris and vulva with his fingers, or using a small vibrator. Relax and allow the sensations of arousal to run through your body. This position is extremely relaxing and can help you to reach orgasm if you are tired and stressed.

Ask your partner to stimulate you with his hands, lips or a vibrator while you lie on your back with your head hanging over the edge of the bed. It is not clear why it works but this position can provide the stimulation needed to tip you over into orgasm. Receiving oral sex while you are in this position is particularly effective.

Imagine yourself having an orgasm. Roll your hips and thrust upwards with your pelvis as if you were experiencing the muscular spasms that occur during an orgasm. As you do this, stimulate yourself by hand or ask your partner to caress you with his fingers or lips.

Read a good sex fantasy book. Try Nancy Friday's *My Secret Garden* or *Women on Top* (available in bookshops or from an Internet site such as www.amazon.co.uk) for help in understanding how fantasy can promote orgasm. Sexual fantasy can make a real difference to your sexual arousal level. Some women feel this is somehow wrong, that they should only concentrate on their partner, but a little fantasy (imagining yourself being seduced or in a passionate sexual encounter) can help you to respond more effectively to your partner.

Try arousing yourself by masturbating with a vibrator or by hand, and then stopping once you begin to feel very aroused. Pause for a while, and then resume arousal. Do this several times until you are highly sexually excited. This 'pause' technique intensifies erotic sensation, allowing you to reach a thrilling climax, and with the greater likelihood of having multiple orgasms.

Painful sex

Sex that is painful falls into two areas: penetration that is possible but very uncomfortable (medically called dyspareunia); or penetration that is impossible (often called vaginismus).

Painful intercourse can ruin your enjoyment of love-making. Some women experience pain only during intercourse, others when being touched. It is crucial that you have a medical check-up to rule out any physical causes of dyspareunia. There are many causes of pain, from infections to scarring and other problems. If you notice the pain when you resume sex after childbirth, make sure you have had a check for any stitches you may have had at the time of the birth. Some medicines (prescription and non-prescription) can add to difficulties. Undiagnosed illnesses can also cause pain on intercourse. For example, some types of diabetes can cause repeated attacks of thrush, making intercourse very painful.

If your health check does not discover any physical cause of pain, try the following:

- *Consider taking up an activity that helps you to relax.* Yoga or another kind of gentle stretching exercise can calm the anxiety that adds to muscle tension, often leading to painful sex.

- *Always use a good lubricant* when your partner stimulates your clitoris or before attempting intercourse. A silicone-based one is best as it lasts longer and creates a 'silky' feeling on the skin. Go to www.emotionalbliss.co.uk for this kind of lubricant.

- ***Ensure that you spend lots of time*** arousing one another before attempting penetration. Avoid sex when you are tired or stressed, and make time for sex when you can relax and enjoy yourself.

- ***Ask your partner*** to run his finger carefully around the entrance to the vagina (using a lubricant), gently stretching the muscles as he does so. Avoid pushing anything into the vagina; just relax as he widens the entrance with his fingers. You can also do this yourself. Regular gentle stretching will help you to feel more confident about penetration.

Vaginismus is a spasm of the muscles at the entrance to the vagina. It is usually caused by tension, and can be extremely painful. It effectively blocks penetration by almost anything – fingers, tampons or a penis. However, there are degrees of vaginismus, so you might be able to use a tampon, but not tolerate a penis. The muscle spasm is out of your conscious control so it is no good a partner telling you to 'just stop doing it' because it originates in your subconscious.

If you experience vaginismus, you should first see your GP. Rarely, problems with a thick or unbroken hymen can cause problems with penetration, as can swelling or infection in the vagina. If this is the cause, your GP will be able to recommend treatment. If your medical check does not find any physical problem, you need to see a psychosexual therapist to help you unblock the anxiety to allow penetration. Vaginismus might always have been present (the first time you attempt intercourse or to insert a tampon, for example) or appear after a traumatic event (rape or a clumsily handled attempt at first intercourse, for example). It is also influenced by the messages your family might have given you about sex, and ignorance of your own body. If you feel that your family influenced you so that sex was seen as 'a bad thing' or that you know little about your body, especially your vagina and genitals, take steps to discover more. Read about sex and sexuality (try *The Relate Guide to Sex in Loving Relationships* by Sarah Litvinoff, 2001) or look for booklets on the subject at your local health clinic. If you want to start a family and vaginismus is preventing this happening, try talking to a midwife about it. Nevertheless, seeing a psychosexual therapist could be the key to unlocking this problem. Find one at the British Association for Sexual and Relationship Therapists (www.basrt.org.uk) or Relate (Yellow Pages under 'Counselling/Advice' or www.relate.org.uk).

Case Study catch up

Paul and April talked through how they could alter their personal stress triggers. Paul agreed to talk to his boss about altering his hours and April decided to take some time during the week for herself. They redecorated their bedroom and chose some new fabrics and lighting that made going to bed feel inviting, rather than yet another place that needed sorting out. They also had a 'sensual weekend' when they undertook sensual activities, eating favourite foods, bathing in the whirlpool tub at their local leisure centre and giving one another massages. They realised that they had allowed their sex life to become a drain rather than a renewal of their relationship. April and Paul took the joint decision to cut up their store cards, and these steps gave them the new start they wanted.

De-stress sex overnight

The ideas in reducing stress listed above will take time to put into practice. After all, it usually takes months to get into a position of chronic stress, so undoing it will also take weeks or months. But you can use the following ideas to make an instant change to your sex life if you feel it is under pressure:

- *Stop the head/body split*. As you start to make love, allow your body to speak to you. Concentrate on the sensations from your skin. If you find yourself thinking negatively, replace the thoughts with positive images and messages.

- *Tell your partner what you want*. If you are rushing through sex it is easy to think 'I'll just do whatever he or she wants'. This raises stress levels because you can start to feel resentful. Break this habit by saying 'touch me here' or 'that feels so sexy'.

- *Allow more time for sex*. Rushed sex (see also Chapter 2, Self-esteem) can cause stress rather than reducing it. Go to bed half an hour earlier, turn off the TV so you can cuddle up without distraction or put aside a whole evening for love-making.

- *Use a good massage oil and/or lubricant during love-making*. Improving the way that your hands slide over skin can have an almost magical effect on love-making because it allows you both to luxuriate in the sensations. Touching also releases feel-good chemicals in the brain, helping to counteract stress.

- *Play relaxing music while you make love*. Slow, dreamy music is proven to alter and slow brainwaves. This will allow you to feel you have all the time in the world to make love, lengthening the time you have to enjoy stimulating one another.

- **See sex as a way of avoiding stress**. Sex aids relaxation, but lots of people see it as an extra stress in their life. If you feel this way, concentrate on the feeling of closeness to your partner that often follows good love-making. Improve the quality of your sex and you will find that sex acts as a preventive to stress, rather than as a cause of stress.

KEY MESSAGE

Remove stress and you will speedily improve your sex life. Remember, sex can help to relax you and prevent stress.

CHAPTER 5

power games

· ·

Sex and power have always been inextricably linked. Powerful people often exude sexual charisma as far as less powerful individuals are concerned. Equally, sexy people usually find they can exert considerable power over others.

History is littered with stories of great men (usually men, as they tended to be the ones with power) who were held in sway by sexually powerful women. Kings of England in particular were susceptible to feminine sexual allure: Henry VIII, who renounced the Catholic Church for Anne Boleyn, and King Edward VIII, who gave up the throne itself for Wallis Simpson, are two of the better documented ones.

Power and fame

Even run-of-the-mill politicians with only a modicum of power end up regularly on the front pages of tabloid newspapers having been caught up in sexual shenanigans with an array of lovers and mistresses. Power and fame probably rank as equal aphrodisiacs, which is why one wit rather cruelly described politics as Hollywood for ugly people.

Most of us don't necessarily wield a great deal of power in society, but being in a couple relationship gives you a huge amount of power over one other person. And although we may like to think we use this power responsibly, when it comes to sex we are probably most likely to set off on a power trip at the expense of our partner.

Sex is about vulnerability. A good sexual relationship with another person allows us to express who we truly are. But by removing our protective outer shell in order to be intimate with someone, it is easier to be hurt and it is easier for us to hurt our partner, even unwittingly, once they have exposed their vulnerability to us.

Sexual power games

You could be forgiven if the phrase 'sexual power games' sounds like it has little to do with you. Quite possibly it brings to mind a couple playing sado-masochistic rituals that involve one partner dominating or even beating their partner for their mutual pleasure and sexual satisfaction. While this is undoubtedly one form of sexual power game, it is a different genre entirely from the more usual sort of power games that occur in couple relationships.

Although extreme forms of sado-masochistic role-playing are the choice of relatively few people, if both partners are happy to abide by a clear set of rules and derive pleasure from it, it does have the advantage of the couple understanding the nature of the game they are playing.

Women who ration sex

Sexual power games stray into damaging territory when they are enacted by couples who don't even realise they are playing a game. Women who ration sex, for example, are playing a power game that is capable of being self-destructive and hurtful to their partners. Two thousand years ago, the Greek playwright Aristophanes wrote a challenging comedy, *Lysistrata*, about women who withheld sex to prevent their men from going to war and, historically speaking, the decision to grant sex was one of the very few real powers that women had.

Frequently, it is still the woman who sets the sexual pace for the couple. These days there are few women who use sex as a form of bartering for material goods (plenty of 1960s housewives were under the impression it was fine to grant sex in exchange for a new fridge), but many still find themselves tempted to withhold sex when they feel angry or overlooked by their partners in other ways.

Sex as a bargaining tool

The effect of denying sex as a punishment, or using it unconsciously as a bargaining tool is twofold. Firstly, it destroys the emotional intimacy that a mutually giving sexual relationship can build between you. Secondly, sooner or later it wrecks the woman's potential for enjoying sex on other occasions. Think about it. By withholding sex as a punishment you are implying that sex is something that matters to your partner, but not to you – or why would you be punishing yourself?

It also means that when a withholding woman does have sex, she often unconsciously feels that she should not act as though she is enjoying it. For if she does, there is a chance that her partner might be tempted to pull the same trick on her on another occasion to express *his* anger or upset.

There is, of course, a significant difference between straightening out a source of conflict between you before you feel ready to make love, and turning your back on your partner to reject them because you are angry with them in some way. If you are a woman who denies her partner sex when you are unhappy with him, take a few moments to think about what sex means to you and to him.

Good sex cements long-term relationships

If refusing sex is an easy way to express your anger with your partner, because you don't much like sex anyway, it may seem like an easy option to take. But be warned. Good sex can be the glue that cements long-term relationships; using sex as a weapon is destructive not just to your sex life but also to your union as a whole.

If you want your relationship to flourish, tackle your negative feelings about sex rather than looking for ways of escaping it. The first step is to talk to your partner in a non-threatening way about your situation. It may simply be that you have become bored with the routine of love-making, or it may be that your partner needs to support you in other areas of your life. Give him or her the opportunity to put things right, rather than meting out the punishment first. (Read more about anger and sex in Chapter 6.)

Giving men power they don't want

And while we are focusing on women, let's look briefly at the (usually female) tendency to hand over responsibility for their sexual satisfaction to their partner. This is giving men a power that the majority of them don't want. That is not to say that they don't want their partners to have a good time. They do. But always taking sole responsibility for someone else's sexual pleasure is too much for even the most skilled and considerate lover. Far too often, women blame men for being a let-down in bed, and accept no responsibility for this themselves.

Try thinking about it this way. If you would not expect a man to choose what you are going to eat in a restaurant, you should not expect him to assume sole responsibility for your sexual satisfaction. But a remarkable number of otherwise articulate and emotionally literate women become mutes the minute they get into bed with a man. And, even worse, they blame their partner for being selfish and not doing enough to please them if they don't have a good time. Men are not mind-readers and every woman has a unique sexual response. A man may be exhausting himself doing something a previous partner adored, but if it leaves you cold and you would prefer something else, *you need to say so.*

Three responsibilities

Both sexes have at least three responsibilities when it comes to sex. The first is to find out what they personally like, and the second is to communicate this important information in a sensitive and non-threatening way. The third responsibility is to act on it.

If you want to try something dramatically or even slightly different in your sex life, talk about it before you begin to make love. Find a quiet, neutral space to mull it over with your partner before you spring your big idea on them. They may be thrilled beyond belief that you want them to dress up as a firefighter/policewoman/stripper, but you must give them a chance to respond to your idea outside the pressure of the bedroom, and possibly offer a few ideas of their own as well.

Sex as a joint venture

If you can always think of sex as a joint venture, and not as something one partner does to the other, then your chances of ending up playing unintentional power games are greatly reduced. The opposite of a man who doesn't seem too aware of his partner's sexual response is the man who gets obsessed with the amount of pleasure he is giving his partner. This is the kind of man who cannot rest unless his partner has at least one orgasm, preferably half a dozen. Although this approach can be appealing initially for a woman, it can soon become exhausting, because the focus is not truly on her, it is on *his* performance. He wants to earn points for giving her a good time, because it confirms his prowess as a lover.

This sort of insecurity needs to be dealt with before it becomes an issue that threatens the couple. It can lead to a woman faking pleasure, simply to keep her partner quiet, and sooner or later this unwanted pressure will affect the quality of the relationship. Once a man can understand that orgasms are not like goals in a football match – a measure of achievement – but rather an enjoyable destination in what should be an entirely pleasurable journey, he can begin to see sex differently, and remove some self-inflicted pressure from his own shoulders at the same time.

Reduce the scope for point scoring

The longer your relationship lasts, the greater the scope for negative point scoring off each other (using sex as your game-card). This is because making love with your partner after the first heady days of infatuation are over is increasingly a decision rather than an impulse. If you have become caught up in calculating whether or not to have sex, and you are basing your decision on anything other than a desire to bring your partner love and pleasure, then you have started, almost imperceptibly, to slide down a road that can become increasingly dangerous.

It is a route that can lead to a vicious cycle of rejection, hurt, refusal and more hurt, and it is possible to get to a place in a relationship where if one of you wants to make love, the other does not, almost as a point of principle. For some people, this is a state of desolation that can last for months or even years.

This destructive pattern is more likely to occur if either of you is lacking in sexual confidence. A woman who is unsure of her attractiveness, for example, will take a 'no' from her husband as a hint that he no longer fancies her. The fact that he is tired, worried or he has just eaten too much supper will pass her by. Similarly, a man who is possibly feeling put down at work may feel humiliated when his wife or girlfriend turns down the opportunity to make love with him. He may take her 'no' as an attack on his masculinity, ignoring the fact that she may be worried about her own job, or be preoccupied with a family difficulty.

A refusal is simply that – one refusal – and it is much more likely to be part of something that your partner is going through than anything to do with you. Of course, if it happens frequently, it is important to establish why you are being turned down. This should not be a third-degree interrogation, but a conversation initiated when you are both feeling relatively calm and you are in an appropriate space together. It may simply be that your partner is seeking reassurance about your feelings for them, or they may be wrestling with a problem they haven't yet been able to discuss with you. Patience and an inclination to listen without judging them or expressing bitter disappointment in their behaviour will get you a long way.

(Building sexual security is discussed in Chapter 8, Trust and Security, but there are some suggestions at the end of this chapter that will help you replace power games with an emotionally healthier approach to your relationship.)

Pornography

The impact of pornography on a relationship is not a subject talked about at length in sex books. Usually there is advice to try it and see if it spices up a flagging sex life, and that's about it. While there are some women who claim to enjoy pornographic films and magazines, generally they are purchased by men.

The reality is that pornography makes a lot of women feel uncomfortable, especially if they sense they are being compared unfavourably to the models in the magazines or movies.

The attraction of pornography is that it gives the user complete control over their sexual experience. They aren't required to make conversation, an effort to please or even a post-coital cup of tea. Men can also indulge fantasies that they may feel unable to discuss with their partner. In small doses, this is probably pretty harmless; the problem for couples arises when it becomes addictive for the man and he is unable to function sexually without it.

If your partnership is troubled by an unhealthy addiction to pornography – and 'unhealthy' means that you can't have a respectful dialogue about it – there may be some deep-rooted underlying issues in your relationship that may be hard for you to sort out by yourselves. Couple counselling, which will give you a neutral space to explore the influences on your sexuality, can help you both sort out your thoughts about a problem that, if unchecked, can eventually split relationships.

Fun power games

Not all power games are damaging to a relationship. Some can be great fun. Bearing in mind that a partnership needs five positive experiences for every one negative one in order to be stable, with a relatively small amount of effort you can introduce some excitement into a previously routine sex life that may set sparks flying. For example:

Seduce your partner

Do you remember the days when your partner seduced you? When there was a frisson to the evening explained by the fact that neither of you were quite sure whether or not you would end up in bed together?

It may seem a very long time ago, especially if it has been replaced by one of you turning to the other at 11.00 at night when you are both exhausted and muttering 'fancy a shag?' What people tend to forget as the years go by is that seduction was not the dull routine you had to go through to get to the exciting part – the sex – *it was the act of seduction that made the sex exciting*.

After all, as most couples who have been together a long time know, sex can be the equivalent of a genital sneeze, and be about as exciting as that sounds. While there may be nothing wrong with such a low-level thrill occasionally, if this is all that your sex life amounts to, you might probably be tempted to abandon it entirely. And, frankly, no one could blame you.

Seducing your partner is an enjoyable and positive power game. It allows you to take control of the circumstances surrounding your love-making, and to exert as much love, charm and sexiness as you can in order to win them over for a spot of wild (or even not-so-wild) passion. If you feel yourself starting to balk at this idea and thinking, 'I've been with my partner for ages, why should I have to make an effort?', remember that this is a two-way street.

In any fulfilling relationship, effort is usually matched with effort, so by instigating a plan of gentle seduction, you may be pleasantly surprised by the response from your partner (especially if you are a man). Generally speaking, women are turned on by what is in their heads: by the words they hear and the actions they see. And as they spend so much of their lives taking care of other people, it is a rare woman who does not appreciate being taken care of herself from time to time.

Really this is what seduction is about. It is saying to another person, 'You are special to me, I want to make an effort for you because, in the words of the L'Oreal advert, you are worth it.' If the last time you seduced your partner is lost in the mists of your distant memory, remember the golden rule of seduction: it does not begin at its destination.

Trying to get your partner turned on in bed five minutes before you want to pounce is not seduction. It is called having a shag. This is all well and good if it works every time for both of you, but if it does not, and you'd like a little more variety, then it is time to consider other options.

There is a school of thought that says the sexual act begins 24 hours before you make love. Although few of us get the chance to plan an entire day around the prospect of sex (after all, we do have to wash the dishes and go to the supermarket, at least), it is worth sticking with the philosophy of preparing for something special.

Six secrets of successful seduction

If you are looking for inspiration, consider the six secrets of a successful seduction below:

1. Think about the location

Pay attention to where you want to make love. If the location is your bedroom, tidy away piles of dirty clothes, turn off the TV and computer and get rid of the chipped coffee mug on the bedside table. The best sex happens when there aren't numerous other distractions; you need to focus on each other and on what you are feeling.

Turn off the overhead light bulb, switch to a couple of lamps or consider lighting some candles instead. Ideally, use the scented variety as they will awaken your sense of smell, and by stirring all your senses you will heighten the sexual experience. (Check scented candles out carefully first, though. Some are delicious, but others smell like chemical lavatory cleaners, so be careful what you buy. Also remember never to leave lighted candles unattended.)

2. Music increases relaxation and sensuality

Think about the sounds that surround you. What we hear has an impact on our body chemistry. Music can alter brainwaves and increase feelings of relaxation and sensuality. Choose the music you know your partner likes, especially if it has good memories or associations for both of you.

3. Begin the seduction early

You may want to begin your seduction long before you reach the bedroom by spending some time having fun elsewhere. A trip to the cinema can work well (choose your film carefully, ideally something light or sexy that you'll both enjoy).

Try visiting an art gallery. (Avoid anything contemporary that's likely to feature maggots or dead sheep.) A study of 2,000 visitors to art galleries by the Institute of Psychoanalytical Psychiatry in Rome showed that a visit to an art museum, or even a church, 'stimulates the erotic senses'. At least a fifth of those interviewed had been so excited by what they saw that they either had a 'fleeting but intense erotic adventure' with someone they had not met before, or, if already accompanied, had experienced an 'amorous upsurge' involving 'unexpected experimentation'.

Art galleries have long been a popular place to meet people, but according to the Italian report, it wasn't just the opportunity of meeting a fellow art lover that appealed to the visitors. It was the excitement of being surrounded by the stirring beauty of the works of art themselves that awakened sexual excitement in the onlookers. So a visit to an art gallery isn't just an intellectual activity. It's a way of waking up your eyes to fabulous objects. And if you are female and over a size 12, it's a delightful reminder that inspiring and beautiful women come in every shape and size.

Remember, too, that for most of us the ideal time to have sex is during the afternoon, when our sex hormones are at their peak. If you are looking to rekindle your sex life, don't assume that you have to wait until it gets dark before you can make love. Build up to making love in the afternoon when hormones are on your side and neither of you are as physically tired as you will be by the end of the day. One weekend, get the children to visit friends and don't invite anyone for Sunday lunch. Give yourselves at least a couple of hours on your own. (If you both work from home or you are retired, sex in the afternoon is a great way to brighten up a dull Monday.)

4. Enjoy a light meal

Food can be a great prelude to sex or it can put paid to it quicker than you can say, 'Can we look at the dessert menu, waiter?' This is because food requires digesting and if you eat a heavy meal, the blood will flow to your stomach to aid digestion, leaving you feeling bloated, lethargic and possibly burping – not a good state to be in before you make love. A light meal, on the other hand, encourages good conversation and a sense of sharing; two habits to take with you into the bedroom.

5. Make an effort with clothes

Dressing up for sex might mean 'costume' type clothes: as a nurse, a naughty maid or perhaps a fireman. However, for most of us it means making an effort to look good for our partner in terms of our outer and underwear. At the very least, for men, that means *clean pants and socks*, a fresh shirt and trousers that have recently seen the inside of a washing machine or the dry cleaner's.

If you are a woman who has never strayed beyond big, comfortable knickers and a greying bra, you may be surprised at the amount of fun you can have buying slightly more sexy underwear. While it is generally appreciated a great deal by men, who are primarily stimulated sexually by what they see, women can find that silks and satins are a turn-on for them too, simply because the textures feel so good next to the skin. And bearing in mind that the skin of a woman is ten times more sensitive than that of a man, soft, furry and velvety fabrics can be a beneficial addition to your wardrobe.

6. The importance of hygiene

Finally, a straightforward word about hygiene. Unless you and your partner belong to a tiny sect who savours the smell of body odour, don't expect someone to cover you in kisses if you don't smell good. For most people, poor hygiene is a total turn-off. Shower and brush your teeth *always*. Never wait to be asked. Women, especially, equate a man who is careful about cleanliness with an emotional safety net. It gives her a message that he isn't interested in selfish sex, he is bothered about *her* too.

Let the seduction begin . . .

Defuse power games

Most couples play power games of one kind or another. Our desire to influence the behaviour of others is part of our basic hard-wiring as human beings. From the first cries of a baby asking to be fed, to the woman who tries subtle hints to get her husband to cook her favourite meal, we seek to control or influence others. Mostly this is normal and acceptable. In fact, without these interactions, society as we know it would grind to a halt. But problems can emerge, as Val has demonstrated, when power and control is used to manipulate a partner into behaving in a way that is detrimental to the relationship.

CASE STUDY •

Phillip and Wanda

Phillip and Wanda, both aged 40, have been married for ten years. Phillip is Wanda's second husband after a previous divorce. Phillip has never been married before and they do not have children. They feel reasonably content with their relationship, except for one area: sex. Phillip feels he is manipulated into having the kind of sex that Wanda dictates. He feels he has to wait until Wanda indicates that she wants sex, and then he must offer only the kind of sex that Wanda wants. This usually means the 'missionary' position and the lights off. If Phillip approaches Wanda for love-making, she becomes silent and withdrawn. This can last for days. Any other approach to love-making technique causes Wanda to stop the sexual activity and sleep in the spare room. Phillip has tried numerous ways of avoiding the problems, but they always seem to end up with Wanda holding all the cards. Phillip feels resentful of Wanda's tight hold on their sex life, whereas Wanda feels anxious about sex in general. She avoids any discussion on the issue and can't even think about it without feeling extremely uncomfortable.

Wanda is controlling Phillip and Phillip is trying to break free. Metaphorically speaking, Wanda has a net and Phillip has a knife — Wanda is continually trying to control Phillip while Phillip is always trying to change things. This kind of set-up is emotionally exhausting for any couple, and has left Phillip and Wanda with a relationship that is slowly being poisoned by a power game.

Wanda has evolved this sexual response partly because of her first marriage. Her ex-husband, Steve, often demanded sex and treated Wanda more as a sex object than a person. She felt out of control around sex and found it difficult to stop Steve getting his way. A year into their marriage Wanda discovered he had been seeing a prostitute and divorced him. She has told Phillip some of this, but still feels the need to remain in control during sex with him. Her unconscious fear is that if Phillip gains any leeway at all he will repeat Steve's abusive behaviour, even though logically she knows that this is unlikely. Wanda and Phillip are caught in a power game that has its roots in Wanda's past.

In control or out of control?

Most sexual power games stem from a desire to control a situation. It may be directly related to sex – you don't want him to see your large bottom so you refuse all positions that show your bum – or unrelated – you are cross because she belittled you in front of your friends so you refuse to respond to her seduction. In either case you are trying to send a message to your partner by code: understand my silence/non-response/refusal to move around in sex and you will know why I feel the way I do. Of course, what usually happens is that your partner is mystified. They may know you are trying to tell them something, but what is it? For example, if you insist on adopting only one position for sex, like Wanda, you could be saying a variety of things. You might be saying that this is the only position that gives you pleasure. Alternatively, that you have a bad back and cannot move around. Or, that there is a cold draught from the window if you move to a different part of the room. Your aim to control the sexual scene actually leaves you both out of control because neither of you is giving, nor receiving, an accurate message.

Why are you playing a power game?

Here are some common reasons for playing power games. Do you identify with any of them?

You feel embarrassed to raise the issue about which you are concerned. For example, you want your partner to give you oral sex more often, but you find it difficult to say this. When you have sex that does not include oral sex, you avoid any sexual advance from them for a few days.

Solve this problem. Many people feel embarrassed to talk about sex. This is surprising given the amount of sexual imagery all around us, but talking to a partner is like learning a language that you both have to create. If you never work out the right words for the two of you, it's no wonder that saying anything is difficult. So, if you want good sex, you need to give voice to your desires. Next time you make love ask for what pleases you. You can do this by encouraging your lover with feelgood groans, placing their hand on the part of the body you want stroked or telling them what you want. For example, Jill told her boyfriend, Sean, that she loved it when he 'licked and kissed' her nipples. Try whispering these feelings in your lover's ear during love-making, lowering your voice to a sultry tone. If you feel comfortable, use earthy words (often called 'talking dirty') to arouse you and your partner. Start with something mild or you might frighten your partner by calling them something they find offensive.

You want to make a point. For example, you have argued over the choice of a new car. Your partner wants a more expensive style while you want an economic run-around. You avoid, and turn down, sex for a while so that they realise how serious you are about your point of view.

Solve this problem. If you are holding out on your partner in this way then you need to settle your disputes outside the bedroom. Talk about any difficulties as they arise rather than hope he or she comes round to your way of thinking.

If you find that discussions get heated, you can use sex to reunite. Avoid doing this in order to shut your partner up – only make up in bed if the problem is almost completely sorted out. Making-up sex can be a heady experience, so here are some ideas to allow it to be even more exciting:

- Take your partner by the hand and lead them to the place you want to make love. This could be your bed, lounge floor or kitchen table! Kiss them on their neck, eyelids, and lips.

- Slowly undress them. Take your time over each button and zip, encouraging them to do the same for you. Slide your hand under their clothes, letting your fingers linger on the warm skin. Stroke the sides of the body (from armpit to hip) in long, firm strokes.

● Gently push them on to the bed or floor (place cushions on the floor first to avoid accidents!), and cover them with your whole body. Look into their eyes and kiss them on the lips, chest, and stomach, savouring each kiss.

● Remove their underwear, but first slide your hands under the material, teasing their genitals or breasts. Run a finger along the groove between the top of the leg and the groin. This area has many responsive nerve endings and feels very erotic when stroked.

● Penetrate (if you are the man) your partner slowly after lots of stimulation by hand and lips on the clitoris. If you are the woman, guide your partner's penis inside you after plenty of time spent caressing his penis.

You want him or her to do what you want. For example, you 'reward' your partner with sex or particular sexual behaviour (a special position or activity that you usually avoid) in order to get him or her to give you what you want. This might be a consumer item or something less tangible, such as agreeing to help a member of the family with a problem.

Solve this problem. Using sex to get what you want could suggest that you keep yourself in reserve, avoiding adventurous sex at other times. It could be that the game element has taken over your response, rather than your ability to tune in to your partner. To prevent this happening, and to break the habit of using sex in this way, try the following:

● As you caress one another during love-making, try to retain eye contact. Most people shut their eyes during sex, but if you try to look at your partner as much as possible, you could find it allows you to connect and stop seeing sex as a persuader for some other means. Listen to what your partner is saying to you during love-making, and respond to their remarks. Compliment them on their body. Tell them how beautiful/handsome they are, and let them know that their body really turns you on.

● Asking him or her to take charge during sex can also help. Try wearing a loose blindfold as a part of sexual arousal as your partner caresses and arouses you, or make a list of the things you both enjoy during love-making and ask him to surprise you with these during sex. Playing a role (cavegirl or caveman, sexy waiter or waitress, lap dancer or stripper, for example) can also be fun, but be careful that this does not become part of a 'reward' for something he has done that pleased you.

You want to avoid responsibility for sex. If you feel under pressure to 'perform' – get sex just right – you may try to pass the responsibility to your partner by never initiating sex or talking about what you like. In this way, you can 'pass the buck' for sexual success to your partner and avoid any blame if love-making does not work out.

Solve this problem. Avoiding responsibility for sex may be happening because you find it difficult to decide what you like. Or you may lack confidence about your own sexual response. You can help to manage this problem by suggesting to your partner that you take turns to initiate sex, or initiate it when your partner is least expecting it (but remember that you still need time and privacy for sex). Try leaving a text message on their phone – perhaps with 'Tonight?' or 'Can't wait for tonight' to tempt their interest. Experiment with taking some control back by dressing for sex – pretty underwear or tight boxer shorts, sexy nightwear or even some attractive jewellery. The naked body, adorned with just a chain necklace or bracelets (if you are a woman) or a subtle sheen of silver at the neck (if you are a man) can be highly arousing, as the contrast between nudity and gold or silver highlights your skin and hair. Taking back some element of your sexuality, however small, can help you feel less dependent on, or demanding of, your partner.

You fear passing control to your partner. If you identify with this item, it is likely that you have been hurt in some way. If you allowed yourself to be vulnerable and open with a sexual partner in the past, and he or she rewarded you by being insensitive and hurtful, you may unconsciously seek to hang on to all the control in love-making. This can happen in various ways. For example, you may choose to make love only in a certain room, only in bed or only at a certain time. You could insist on wearing certain items of clothing or that your partner wears something special. And you may want lights on or off, silence or conversation, eyes open or closed. Whatever happens, you need a certain degree of control to feel emotionally safe.

Solve this problem. Controlling what happens during love-making can kill eroticism and creativity. Prevent this kind of behaviour by choosing a room or time to make love that you would normally avoid. Ask your partner where they would like to try making love. For example, try the shower or bathroom for sensuous water play (use the water as a lubricant for caresses and stimulation), the kitchen for sitting on worktops. If you are a woman, sit on the worktop with your legs apart so that your partner can stand between your thighs and enter your vagina. (He may need a stool to reach the right height.) Or use the lounge so you can use the soft chairs and sofas while you experiment with different sexual positions.

Ask your partner to choose one thing he or she really loves and offer to include it the next three times you make love. You could also ask him or her to show you exactly how they like their clitoris or penis to be stimulated, and then spend some time learning their 'technique'. This will need a little patience, but sharing what turns you both on and taking a few steps outside of your 'comfort zone' will enable you to feel less burdened by control in sex.

Preventing power games

Ultimately, power games damage relationships. They can become more and more complicated, confusing both of you and hurting whichever partner is on the receiving end. They also beget more games – she withholds sex so he stays out with the lads until the early hours; he demands sex 'doggy style' so she secretly overspends on the credit card to comfort herself for doing something she doesn't want and to punish him for his request.

Here is how to prevent these damaging games:

Improve your self-esteem

Chapter 2 outlines boosting self-esteem and will help you to stop playing this kind of game. If you feel good about yourself, you do not need to manipulate others into doing what you want. For example, if you shut down sex because you think this is the only way your partner will notice you are upset or annoyed, then you lack the self-confidence to explain how you feel.

Analyse why you play the game

Are you afraid of the outcome if you raise the issue you are concerned about? Do you secretly fear your partner will not listen to you if you tell them how you feel? Have you had experience of your partner riding roughshod over your feelings so your 'game' acts as a defence? Try writing down what you think your feeling(s) would be if you stopped the game and tried to be straightforward. For example, is it fear, anger, sadness, anxiety or another feeling? These are the feelings you are trying to avoid. Facing these thoughts could help you develop the courage to stop playing your particular game.

Explain why you want to stop the game

Most games take more than one player. You may want to stop, but if your partner has been part of the game for a long time, they will need to know that you want things to be different. For example, Marie had this problem with her partner, Roger. She wanted him to stop drinking heavily and decided to say, 'I wonder if you have noticed that when you go out and get drunk on a Saturday night I put a stop on sex for some time afterwards. This is because I think you don't listen when I say how much your drinking upsets me. I know you don't do it all the time, but I often feel threatened by your behaviour. I will agree to stop using sex as a punishment if you will meet me halfway and agree to avoid drinking so heavily.'

In this example, Marie has been clear about why she has previously tried to use sex to change Roger's drinking, but also promised to change if Roger will alter his behaviour. They will both need to make some compromises, but they have a degree of equality in these and this will help. Marie is also non-accusatory, enabling Roger to respond without being upset. Try writing down what you want to say.

It is not easy to counteract years of using sex for other reasons, so be gentle on yourself. If you can't get it all sorted in one go, just keep going until you have both managed to make sense of what you want.

Teach yourself 'sex speak'

The chief cause of game playing in sex is lack of effective communication. If you find you can't say that you like/dislike a certain sexual activity or want to make a change to your sex life, then you will end up speaking in code – either by denying sex or trading sex for something else.

Use positive rather than negative remarks

Say 'I love it when you touch me here' rather than 'I've told you a hundred times, stop doing that and touch me here.' Take their hand and guide them to the spot you want caressed. Do this gently and with understanding, without a show of exasperation.

If you are too tired or cross, say so

Some couples play a complicated game where they try to outdo one another in making love whatever the underlying feelings sparking between them. If you have real reasons why sex is not on your menu, explain. Make it clear you are not rejecting them as a person, only the sex act at that time. If you have a row, try to settle it outside of the bedroom before it eats away at your sex life.

Feed back what you are feeling

If you think your partner ought to know by mind-reading what is pleasing you, it's time to give up on telepathy. You don't need to deliver an essay on his or her technique. Use lots of 'mmm's', 'aaah's' and 'yes, yes, yes!' to get your message across. Most couples find that sexual communication enhances sex rather than diminishes enjoyment.

Be honest about what you like

If you really hate something that your partner suggests, it is better to say 'That really doesn't turn me on' than go along with his or her suggestion and store it for payback on something else later. Look for win/win suggestions. For example, say, 'I don't enjoy dressing up as a maid, even though it arouses you, but I am willing to buy some sensuous underwear to flaunt for you.' Or offer to do something they enjoy in return for something you love. But you should never feel pressurised into an activity you feel uncomfortable or degraded by.

Your guide to using porn together

The debate about pornography centres on whether the people who appear in pornographic magazines, videos and films are being used or abused, or take part because it is their chosen lifestyle and job.

One side of the argument states that people, and especially women, are demeaned by appearing in pornography, chiefly because more men than women use porn and women become objects rather than living, breathing humans. The other side says that many porn stars are paid thousands for their 'acting' and we should accept this in the same way that we accept Hollywood actors playing a role. Whichever side of the divide you think you are on, it is likely that you have considered using some kind of porn to boost your sex life. It is a tricky subject, but if you feel it is not for you, then don't feel you should make yourself look at porn imagery or read soft-porn books or magazines. It is OK to say no, even if your partner is more interested than you are.

The reason I am including porn in this section is that many power games centre on sexual experimentation. Your partner may want you to watch a sexy video, but you feel embarrassed or ashamed at the thought of it. Alternatively, you may want to share a sexy scene from a novel, but think your partner may see it as a sign to introduce harder porn into your love life. However, using porn, and avoiding power games, can be done. Here are some guidelines you can follow. Remember that women are turned on more by sound and words than images. Men seem to respond more to films and sexual suggestion in diagrams and photos.

If you are a woman, try reading some erotic books. Great literature contains quite a lot of erotic material (D.H. Lawrence's *Lady Chatterley's Lover* and Nabokov's *Lolita*, for example), so peruse the shelves at your library for unexpected sex scenes in well-known literature. You could also experiment by reading any of the erotic novels, many of which are written for women, that are now on sale in bookshops. (The publishers Black Lace produce this kind of material.) Sexual fantasy also appears regularly in *Cosmopolitan* magazine, and in some other women's monthly publications. *In the Buff* magazine appears on www.emotional bliss.co.uk. This website is safe, but be careful where you surf. Many porn websites are extremely offensive and illegal.

If you want to try a soft-porn video, visit a reputable website that sells only legal material. Try www.passion8.com for sexy DVDs and videos to buy. You can also rent this kind of video, but you may feel embarrassed about taking one out from your local Blockbusters! You may find it more acceptable to watch one of the *Lovers' Guide* videos that are available to buy from high street stores. These videos show graphic sex scenes, but are aimed at helping you to enjoy love-making more and have an educational slant. Women tend to find this kind of video more acceptable.

Some couples find it arousing to look at sexy magazines together, but you need to decide what level of magazine you both feel comfortable with. Some mainstream men's magazines (*FHM* and *Loaded*, for example) contain raunchy pictures that could act as a turn-on, but many of these are intended to stimulate men rather than women. There are some sexy magazines available for women, but you need to search for them. Try reading *The Erotic Review* (www.theeroticreview.com) for tasteful but explicit sex scenes and stories suitable for men and women.

If you decide you want to use porn for stimulation during sex you need to consider how and when you will use it. You could use pictures or photos by sitting together in bed and sharing views and opinions on what you are looking at before making love. If you are looking at a soft-porn magazine (a 'lads' mag') you can tell your partner that you want to try what the man/woman in the picture is doing or whisper seductively in your partner's ear that you fancy trying out their position. You might also suggest that you read a section from a sexy book or magazine to your partner, or that they read to you. Using a seductive tone, while sitting naked with them, and describing an arousing scene from a story, could be an explosive start to sex. Videos or DVDs are good as warm-ups, but avoid leaving them running during love-making itself, as you could feel alienated or in competition with the actor on the screen. The best thing is to watch them together, exchanging kisses and intimate caresses, turning them off once you feel sexually excited. If you want to experiment with running the film during sex, try turning the sound off so that the film is not intrusive in your love-making unless you want to pause and watch a scene together. Some people choose themed porn films, often set in a particular time in history such as ancient Rome or Egypt, or King Charles II's court, for example, and dress up to match the film. You could try this by buying a Cleopatra wig, turning a sheet into a toga, or renting a historical costume that you will wear to watch the film. This can be fun, but you both need to agree that it is OK to do this. It is also a million miles away from the seedy 'dirty mac' image of porn that prevents many couples from considering it. The key to using porn in your sex life is to choose a level that you feel comfortable with and to share it as an addition to your love life, rather than making it the focus of sex.

If you find that porn begins to take over your sex life, or if you or your partner finds it difficult to get aroused without porn, then you need to seek help to deal with this. Your GP may be able to refer you to psychological help, or talk to a therapist listed at the British Association for Sexual and Relationship Therapists (www.basrt.org.uk).

If there are any pre-existing problems that you or your partner are experiencing with using porn, then avoid using it at all during love-making. Unfortunately, sex addiction is on the rise since the Internet brought pornographic imagery into the home at the click of a button. If you want help with porn or sex addiction, contact SA (Sexaholics Anonymous), PO Box 6376, London, N2 0TZ; telephone: 07000 725463.

Case Study catch up

Wanda and Phillip decided to use the ideas from this section to help them overcome their sex power game. Wanda started by writing down what she felt was the reason behind her need to control sex. She then spoke to Phillip about her list. She told him all about the abusive relationship with Steve. This helped Phillip to understand why Wanda felt the way she did. He was able to comfort and reassure her that he would never treat her in this way. Phillip agreed to use positive responses to Wanda as she tried being more experimental in love-making so that she could feel encouraged, and to boost her self-esteem. They also took things in steps. Rather than trying to change everything overnight, they changed one thing each time they made love – leaving the light on, changing positions during sex and so on. Over the coming months, they found themselves enjoying sex. Wanda was less afraid and Phillip felt freer. This gave them the confidence to experiment with what they wanted in love-making, creating a virtuous circle where positive experiences led to greater confidence.

Stop power games tonight

- *Ask yourself why you are playing the game*. Who really wins if you are both unhappy as a result?

- *Be honest about your feelings*. Manipulating your partner by lying or silence is no way to create a loving relationship.

- *Give your partner straightforward feedback* about what you like/dislike in bed. Don't criticise or demean them. Just say what you want in a loving way.

- *Believe in yourself*. If you feel your partner holds all the cards you may try to gain power by playing a game – withholding or trading sex. A high sense of self-esteem will prevent you trying to gain power in this underhand way.

- *Stop holding grudges*. Feeling miffed for a month because he bought a bunch of flowers from a garage on his way home from work for your anniversary when you wanted a posh meal out is a waste of emotional energy.

● ***Stop thinking he or she should know what you want in bed***. Love does not give you telepathic skills. Say or show them during love-making so they understand.

● ***Allow yourself to think about what you need rather than what you want***. For example, you may think you *want* sex with all the bells on, when what you really *need* is sex that satisfies your physical and emotional needs by offering love and warmth rather than mere sensation that soon seems empty and meaningless.

● ***Ask yourself why your partner behaves the way they do***. Try to understand where they are coming from. You may not agree with their point of view, but understanding why they feel the way they do could help you unravel the games you play.

● ***Don't accept abusive behaviour***. Sex that is forced or demanded is not love-making. Make sure your partner knows where the line lies if you feel you have been made to under- take sex you dislike. If he or she loves you, they should not ask for sex that demeans you.

● ***Stop trying to control the outcome of sex***. Good sex comes from going with the flow of what is arousing and satisfying, not making sure your partner (or you) behaves in a certain way.

KEY MESSAGE

Power games prevent good sex. Point scoring, trading sex for other things or trying to control a partner through sex destroy intimacy and trust.

anger

· ·

There are some couples who use anger as a form of fore-play. These are the people who claim that the best sex you can have is after an angry row. It is true that for some a blazing argument can lead to passionate 'making up'. This is because some of the side effects of anger, like a flush-ed face and increased heart rate, are similar to those of sexual arousal.

But there are far better ways of injecting excitement into a relationship that are much less likely to rock its foundations in the long term. (A spot of wild dancing or abseiling down a cliff will produce an equivalent adrenaline rush that will stir up your sex drive, and they are guaranteed to bond you together better than an angry row.)

Dealing with anger is one of the hardest jobs to manage in a relationship between two people. This is partly because it is an emotion that tends not to surface until the 'honeymoon' period of being in love is over. When the hormonal cocktail of love chemicals is flooding through your body, the chances are that you find virtually every aspect of your partner endearing, fascinating and charming.

Ironically, the very attributes that you most like to begin with can prove to be the same ones that make you angry as the years go by. A wild and crazy sense of humour, for example, which may seem innovative and fun in the early days, can turn out to be downright irritating when the relationship is no longer about being wacky but about sharing responsibility for a home and children.

How men and women react to anger

Anger is a perfectly natural response to certain life events, but as children we are programmed to deal with it very differently. Often there is a divide between the sexes. Broadly speaking, men are allowed to give vent to anger and women are taught to suppress it.

To an extent, anger is an acceptable emotion for a man to show in society. Quite often men get angry when they are actually experiencing other emotions, like feeling hurt or vulnerable, but showing these feelings is not something they have been encouraged to do. As a result, uncomfortable emotions in a man are more likely to surface as an angry outburst, say, rather than a flood of tears.

This can be hard for their female partners to manage. Faced with an unhappy man, a woman usually wants to offer comfort and support. Faced with an angry man, however, even if that anger is not immediately directed at her, it is a natural instinct for her to want to protect herself from it and move away.

Understanding anger

There are very few women who want to make love to an angry man. If a man can learn to identify and express his other emotions, rather than using anger as a vehicle for them, he will be guaranteed a much warmer response from his female partner.

Women, on the other hand, have often received messages as children that angry little girls are not 'nice' or acceptable. As a result, rather than shouting or exploring their anger, they channel it in other directions, even turning it in on themselves when it manifests as depression (some men do this too).

Anger is not necessarily a 'bad' emotion. Anger can stir you to want to put right an unjust situation in your own life or someone else's; it can move individuals to make changes in society and it can jump-start you into action when previously you may have been slow to make a change for the better in your life. It is also fine to get angry with your partner. Any two people who are creating an interesting and rewarding life together are bound to have disagreements about ideas or issues in their lives. What is essential, though, is to know how to handle anger when it arises.

Conflict is a fact of life. Avoiding it does not mean you have a peaceful life; it means you have a life in which potentially important feelings and experiences are buried under the surface. And it is this buried anger that can begin to gnaw away at your relationship. Sex may be one of the first areas of your life that will begin to be affected by it.

When we are counselling couples, Julia and I often see two individuals who love each other, but who have no blueprint for dealing with conflict in their relationship. Often they will say that they have no memory of their parents ever having a row, or even a minor disagreement.

In reality, the chances are that their parents did not live lives in which nothing bad, difficult or irritating ever happened. They were human beings, after all, and bad, difficult and irritating is part of the human condition. The likelihood is that their parents didn't have a good mechanism for dealing with anger either, and as such one or other parent capitulated whenever an area of conflict came up, creating other, less apparent but still very real difficulties in the relationship. (Probably sexual ones, at the very least.)

Problems also arise when two people come together who have experienced entirely different ways of handling anger in their families. If one person comes from a family that shouts, slams doors and storms about for half an hour before it's all over, it is a big shock to encounter someone whose anger turns them silent, cold and uncommunicative for three days (and vice versa).

An angry woman won't want sex

Few angry women will want to make love. This is because, for most women, an enjoyable sexual relationship involves emotional intimacy and a feeling of closeness. Anger pushes you away from another person, and if you are a man you may find that an approach to have sex made while your female partner is angry with you is met with even more fury on her part.

If you haven't had sex in a long while, and there is no physical reason preventing you, think long and hard about whether there is anger on either side festering in the relationship. In partnerships where there has been no sex for years, sometimes there is a wife who has not been able to forgive her husband for an affair, nor come to terms with her own feelings about it. (Read more about affairs in Chapter 8, Trust and Security.) Sometimes the anger is nothing to do with the partner, but it could be to do with a tragic life event, like losing a child or a beloved parent, causing unresolved anger that is acting as a permanent dampener on desire.

If these ideas seem a long way from the process of getting your sex life back on track, be patient. Rekindling a sex life isn't just about the external stuff like getting in touch with being sensual again and having fun together; it is about what is going on inside your heads too. If you can sort out the mental difficulties that may have been preventing you from connecting sexually with each other, you will be a very long way down the road to building a good sex life together again.

A combination of emotions

When you get angry about something, it is usually because that issue is important to you. It can help if you understand that anger is usually a combination of emotions, rather than one single state. Try thinking of anger as a warning flag that there is an issue that wants your attention. For example, if you receive unfair treatment at the hands of your boss, a certain degree of anger is understandable. That anger might prompt you to seek a meeting to present your concerns, or to take steps that in some way will correct the situation.

If you feel nothing but blind fury, however, and you are inclined to spend hours pondering the most excruciating ways in which you might exact your revenge, it is a different situation. The chances are that (a) resentment has been building up over a series of slights for a long time and you are in the wrong job; (b) your boss represents something bigger for you than simply being the person who oversees your work; or (c) there is something else going on in your life that is deeply troubling you and you have mixed it up with your situation at work.

The emotions underlying these other reasons can be many and varied. They may range from fear that you will lose your job (and end up destitute on the streets – a more common anxiety than you might think), to a disappointment with yourself and an uncomfortable feeling that deep down you are a failure. These feelings don't have to be true, indeed the reverse is often the case, but you have to perceive them as true to be affected by them.

Other sources of anger

Angry feelings can come from other situations in the present and the past, as well as the immediate, which are making us angry. In a sexual relationship, you may find yourself getting angry when your partner unwittingly does or says something that reminds you of a time when you were hurt by a previous lover. In a long-term relationship, you may feel anger when an action or word by a partner sparks a memory of a bad time together, even if it occurred many years before.

Your anger might go even further back, to other unresolved issues from your family life when you were a child. If you come from a large family, for example, and often felt overlooked, you may find it hard to cope with when your usually attentive lover focuses their attention on others at a party, or suddenly becomes caught up with extra work.

It can also be useful to remember that if your partner gets angry with you, it may be because *other* emotions that are *nothing to do with you* are being stirred up for them. It may even be about something that is going on in their life outside your couple relationship. Instead of reacting defensively to protect yourself, it can be more helpful to ask them, in a calm and non-judgemental way, to think about where their anger is coming from.

Look behind the anger

So, if you want to unravel damaging, angry feelings yourself, try looking behind the anger and asking yourself what the emotions are that are making you angry. Is it insecurity, for example, and a worry that your partner might leave you? It's remarkable how many of us express this kind of fear by being unpleasant to our partner, and meting out treatment that is far *more* likely to drive them away from us, rather than sitting down with them and calmly talking it through.

Sometimes people get angry when they 'fall out of love' with their partner and feel disappointed that the romantic hero or heroine they thought had swept them off their feet turns out to be a person with failings and fears themselves. Becoming aware that the person you love is simply a human being with frailties of their own is actually a mature and adult process, it is not necessarily a reason to run off in the opposite direction.

In a long-term partnership, there is always the time when being 'in love' wears off, but what you should be left with is a love that is much richer and longer lasting. After all, although it's easy to be loved by someone whose hormones have decided you seem perfect, it is much more rewarding to be loved by someone who has grown to know who you really are over the years and still loves you, possibly even more than when you first met.

Try thinking of anger as a neutral emotion, which is either helpful or harmful, according to the way you handle it. Anger itself is a normal human response; it need not be the catalyst that means the end of a relationship. Some couples bury anger for years because they are terrified that expressing it will mean the end of everything. This is not a recipe for a happy relationship. Unexpressed anger surfaces in other ways – usually to the detriment of your sexual relationship. This is because sex literally requires us to be naked and physically and emotionally vulnerable, and if we are angry we can find this too much to bear.

What people who bury anger are really frightened of is the wrath caused by anger handled badly. This happens when we attack or blame our partner and make hurtful or sarcastic remarks. It is also when we try to make them feel bad by using negative sentences that begin with 'you' instead of explaining to them how we feel about the issue and using sentences that begin with 'I'.

If you want to approach your partner because your relationship is making you angry and you want to discuss it, try, if you can, to stick to marriage expert John Gottman's suggestions for talking about stress and anger in a marriage:

- *Complain but don't blame*. Avoid phrases like 'It's all your fault' and 'I knew I shouldn't have trusted you.' Just state the problem and describe how it makes *you* feel.

- *Make statements that begin with 'I' instead of 'you'* – this is a vital one. When people hear 'you' before a criticism they feel attacked and defensive. You are not going to get a positive response to your worry from a person who feels threatened.

- *Be clear*. Women especially tend to moan in generalisations, saying things like 'This house is such a mess' and expect their partner to mind-read what they would like them to do about it. Try saying, 'Would you clear your clothes off the bedroom floor, please' and leave it at that. You don't have to add anything to it. It also helps hugely if you are polite when you ask someone to do a task and show your appreciation when they have done it. You don't have to overwhelm them with compliments. Just 'Thanks for doing that' is usually enough.

- *Don't store things up*. If you have been gritting your teeth and saying nothing while getting increasingly angered by aspects of your partner's behaviour, it might be tempting to unleash a torrent of complaints and criticism when you do sit down to talk. Don't. Swallowing back your anger will have caused the most minor transgressions to escalate in your mind, and it is unfair on them if you expect a complete overhaul in their behaviour, having previously not mentioned anything at all.

Explosive, blaming anger is not the only sort that damages relationships. People who sulk can make the lives of those around them very uncomfortable. They are demonstrating a silent anger that allows no chance to resolve the issue and clear the air.

Shouting or silence as a way of handling anger are equally flawed, simply because 'winning' through shutting up your partner with shouting and rage, or getting them to give in because they can't stand being ignored any longer, is at best an incredibly short-term victory. Both behaviours will instil anger or distress in your partner, and neither is conducive to solving the situation that made you angry in the first place.

Expressing anger positively

However, expressing anger in a positive way enables you to overcome difficulties and ventilate feelings that might otherwise end up corroding your relationship. So the key question is: how do you express anger positively?

Firstly, you need to be able to express it cleanly, sticking to how you are feeling and not straying on to the path of blaming or attacking your partner. Refrain from judging the person who you believe to be the source of your anger, and try, if you can, to look inside yourself at what is really pushing your buttons. If you can only see red mist, and the last thing you feel like doing is analysing yourself, try not to do anything at all until you are feeling calmer. This might take ten minutes or an hour. Just let your partner know that you need a little space, but you will be back to deal with the problem. Don't walk away with the implied or stated suggestion that you are turning your back on the whole wretched business.

If you can feel the temperature rise in a conversation and you both begin to get heated, resist the temptation to lash out automatically if your partner says something unkind or tactless. Make yourself wait five minutes before responding. American researchers have found that when people were asked what they'd do if a partner behaved badly, they were more likely to respond destructively if they were asked to give a fast response. A pause of as little as *six seconds* was enough to make them think more constructively, calm down and weigh up the consequences of what they were about to say. So even if you can think of the most tremendous put-down and you are itching to get back at your partner, resist the urge to say it if you care about the future of your relationship.

Follow the guidelines on having a helpful argument below and you may find that anger becomes a useful tool in keeping your relationship on track and your sex life alive.

How to have a helpful argument

Remember that being able to express disagreements between you actually reduces stress in your relationship. Rows which are just about anger and sarcasm clearly do nothing to benefit your relationship, but many couples come adrift because they don't know how to talk to each other when things start to go wrong. As a result, the distance between them widens and they drift further and further apart.

The best rule for having a 'good' row is that neither of you try to come out on top. If one of you ends up feeling victorious, it will mean that the other will end up feeling a loser, and you can guarantee that the victor's glory will be short-lived. If you solve a dispute where you both end up feeling satisfied, you can be pretty sure that the source of the stress that created the original argument will have been satisfactorily dealt with . . . to the relief of both of you.

So here are some suggestions for having a 'good' row:

- Ensure that your arguments are free from any taint of violence or aggression.

- Make sure you are wearing clothes and sitting up. Even if sex is the issue, don't try to solve it while you are naked and lying down together. You will feel more vulnerable than usual and it's best to keep love-making separate from rows (even the healthy, positive variety).

- Keep disagreements contained – make sure they don't go on for hours, or even days, and are satisfactorily resolved in less than 24 hours.

- Even if you are in the middle of a dispute, still try to see things from your partner's point of view.

- Don't use sarcasm, or ridicule your partner or what they are saying.

- When the dust has settled, say sorry for any hurt you have caused.

- Resolve to sort out the cause of your argument. For example, if you have argued about money, sit down one evening and take your finances apart so that you can tackle the source of the dispute.

- Decide a strategy for dealing with the issue that has led to the row.

- Don't drag up the same issue the next time you are in conflict about something else.

- Forgive your partner for any hurt they have caused you.

Untangle anger and sex

As Val has pointed out, anger and sex do not mix. Passion and sex go together brilliantly, but anger and passion are worlds apart. Passion is what you feel when you have a powerful conviction, are swept along by events or overcome with sexual desire. Anger can very occasionally be motivating, but more often it deadens emotions and perceptions. Instead of causing your senses to feel heightened and excited in the way that passion can, the aftermath of anger is often a dull, heavy and 'cut-off' feeling, preventing you from enjoying sex or being open to your partner's needs.

CASE STUDY •

Rhianna and Marcus

Rhianna and Marcus found that anger almost destroyed their sex life. Marcus had always been hot-tempered, even as a child. He was not physically violent, but could shout and yell at Rhianna over what seemed to her to be insignificant issues. Rhianna was no shrinking violet herself, and their arguments often involved extended angry exchanges, slammed doors and remarks that both of them frequently regretted in the cold light of day. They were also bad at saying sorry. They tended to have fierce rows, a couple of days of not speaking and a gradual return to normality – until the next argument. Rhianna and Marcus knew they loved each other, but often felt that their love was stretched to its limits.

Arguments over sex were among the most frequent in their disagreement topics. Rhianna felt that Marcus asked for sex too frequently, that it was too short and that he rolled over to sleep straight afterwards without cuddling her. Marcus felt that Rhianna was withholding and non-experimental during sex. After eight years (the length of time they had cohabited) of rowing they found it almost impossible to initiate sex as it was so fraught with emotional bear traps.

. . . .

If, like Rhianna and Marcus, you know that your sex life can be spoilt by anger, whether it is expressed openly or simmers within, here are some ways of dealing with anger and its effects on your love life.

Taking body action

Before you can deal with the emotional side of anger it is helpful to notice the effect it has on your body and body language. Most anger produces a 'fight or flight' response. Your breathing will speed up, you sweat more and you find it harder to concentrate. If you take some time to work on these physical responses when you start to feel angry, your anger level will decrease and you will find it easier to talk rationally.

If you know you rise to anger quickly, do the following:

Breathe more slowly and deeply. Breathe in through the nose and out through the mouth. Observe your breathing and concentrate on slowing it down.

Look at your partner. Try to maintain eye contact. If possible, remain seated opposite each other.

Try not to shout. Make yourself speak a little slower than usual and avoid blame-making statements such as 'You make me feel . . .' or 'You are totally to blame because . . . '. State what you feel, simply and carefully.

Relax your muscles. Common tension zones are neck, shoulders and back. Let your shoulders relax and your arms hang loosely.

Emotional calming

Arguments over sex are often the most painful a couple can have. This is because you are most vulnerable about being intimate with another. Our ancient ancestors would have got sex over with quickly because while mating any animal is vulnerable to attack. Biologically speaking, sex is distracting and takes us off our guard. It means laying aside our natural defences to allow another human physically close to us. Our thousands of years of civilisation have covered sex in layers of sophistication so that nowadays we do not seek to get mating over with in a few minutes! But the vulnerability of sex remains, so that if we let another person close to us we want to feel reasonably safe with them. If you fight over sex it can threaten this feeling of safety.

Ask yourself the following:

Where does my anger really belong?

Most couples carry anger into other areas of their life at least some of the time. For example, if you are arguing about childcare, you could find it emerges in sex. You may want to withhold sex to drive your message home or push your partner to make love in order to feel in control of a situation outside the bedroom. Work on resolving anything that makes you angry and ends up expressed through your love life. For example, if you resent the fact that your partner never helps with domestic chores, talk to him or her about it and find a way to sort this out. Using sex as a code for 'I'm upset/angry/unhappy about something' doesn't let your partner know what you are really feeling aggrieved about.

Incidentally, money and sex seem to be argument buddies! If you get angry about how your partner behaves around cash, then it can often be played out in bed. This is probably because essentially money is often seen as an exchange in the way that sex is. You give money to receive, save or spend in the way that you might share affections or sexual activity. Therefore, anxieties or annoyances about money can trigger sexual rows and vice versa. Some couples find that if they sort out their financial arrangements their sex rows disappear. Try it and see if money and sex have a hidden link in your relationship.

Do I rely on sex to 'say' everything?

One of the reasons that sex can become such a 'hot potato' is that some people want sex to carry the whole burden of their emotional expression to another. They are often the kind of person who finds it hard to say or show what they are feeling. Sex becomes the only place where they can show their feelings in a socially acceptable way. ('Being intimate in sex is OK because it's what an adult is supposed to do.') In this situation, a refusal from your partner, or a failure of a partner to orgasm, can feel like a devastating personal slight. The pressure on sex in these circumstances can be crushing. Your partner may also unconsciously realise that if they want to get their angry message across, sex is the one place where you will hear it. So they may withhold or reward you with sex. Both of you end up in an emotional desert with sex as a mirage on the horizon.

The best way to deal with this situation is to loosen up and behave more emotionally outside of sex. Talk to your partner about what you are feeling, be demonstrative and warm towards them, and have the occasional row when you feel angry. The more you are able to express yourself naturally, the less the emotional weight on sex. Sex can then become a place to play, to feel passionate and where a refusal or small problem does not take on earth-shattering proportions.

Does working out our anger during sex solve anything?

My bet is that the answer to this question is 'no'. If withdrawing sex because they refused to lend you money, or criticising your partner's sexual technique because they had moaned about a meal you cooked them, really worked you would have a perfect relationship by now! You might get a short-term solution because your partner gets part of the message, but often the whole issue is repressed, only to emerge later because you haven't fully resolved it.

Look at ways of solving disputes without using sex as a battle-ground. For example, if you feel aggrieved because your partner is neglecting you for work, don't take revenge by pretending to 'have a headache' every time he or she asks to make love. Tell them how you feel long before you get to that stage. Trade time together for work, or ask him or her to put aside two evenings a week and one day at the weekend just to be with you. Hoping they understand your unhappiness as you roll over and go to sleep without touching them is unfair and unlikely to get you the attention you want.

Do I expect a mind-reader in bed?

One of the core sources of sexual anger is expecting your partner to know exactly what you need and want to arouse you. Or to understand your reasons for objecting to a particular sexual practice without ever having it explained. For example, when Olivia was 15 she had been hurt by a boyfriend who touched her breasts roughly and with little consideration for her feelings. He behaved as if it was his right to touch Olivia in any way he chose. Later in life, Olivia met Greg. They had a good sex life until Greg tried to caress her breasts. She became tense, and on one occasion told Greg to 'get off' her and climbed out of bed. Greg was mystified about why Olivia behaved this way, but Olivia felt incensed. She thought that if Greg loved her he would realise how she felt about having her breasts touched.

If you feel angry when your partner doesn't deliver the kind of touching you want, you must dispense with the idea that love gives you ESP. Tell them what you like and dislike. Guide their hands over your body, whisper in their ear what you want (usually a great turn on!) or demonstrate by masturbating for them so they can see the tempo and pressure you like. If you want to make love, don't give clues that you hope they will pick up. A well-known divorce case of some years ago saw a man attempt to divorce his wife because he felt she wilfully misunderstood him when he said he was going to have a bath when he was really asking for sex!

Ask in a romantic and loving way – 'I really want you tonight', 'You turn me on – let's go to bed', 'Let's make love' – are all better than 'I'm going to bed now' or 'Let's have an early night', both of which can be misunderstood. If you have private jokes about asking for sex, use them, but only if they do not hurt your partner. Saying 'Let's have a look at this huge bum you're always on about' is not a turn-on! (A friend told me this was actually something her ex-husband said to her. It helped her decide to get a divorce.)

Do I want someone who is constantly sexually available?

Imbalance in sexual desire is a very common couple problem. She wants it, he doesn't, or vice versa. A complex set of games can ensue where one partner accuses the other of sexual disinterest, only to be told they are also withholding. (Look at Chapter 5,

Power Games, for more information on power and sex.) The truth is that research into sexual desire demonstrates that it ebbs and flows throughout the lifetime of a couple. Recent research suggests that women of all ages are on a longer 'desire cycle' (about ten days) than men (about three to five days, although this lengthens as men age). This means that women may want sex less than men, but are capable of feeling desire if not pressed into love-making when they are not ready. Women may also experience responsive desire rather than spontaneous desire. (In essence, women think less about sex but feel desire when approached in a way they feel comfortable about.) All this means that if you want a mature and loving relationship you need to negotiate on when and how often you make love. Sulking because your partner has turned you down only increases the pressure your partner feels, making sex less likely. If your partner rejects sex, they are not rejecting you, only the act on that occasion. Be affectionate and loving and ask again another time.

Your guide to injecting sexual excitement

Sexual boredom is an issue that strikes most couples once their relationship is established. The thrill of meeting when you are both new to each other can lend sex a feeling of excitement that appears to decline once you have been together for a while. This can lead to arguments because you or your partner may seek to place blame for the lack of sparkle during sex. Experimenting with different sexual activities can greatly help you to avoid sexual boredom and prevent the arguments that originate from the feeling that all the spice has left your relationship. Here are some ideas to encourage you to feel more interest and excitement during sex. You may not want to try all the suggestions, but just one or two could make all the difference to your love life:

Who are you pleasing?

Stop trying to please only your partner. I know – you thought caring, loving sex was about making your partner happy. Yes, this is true. You do need to help your partner to feel fulfilled during lovemaking. Pretending they do not exist in order to get your own satisfaction is a recipe for sexual problems. Nevertheless, if you think back to how you felt when you first got together, chances are that the thrills you experienced when anticipating sex were about your own sexual desire, not your partner's. The problem with committed relationships is that many couples become focused on pleasing their partner, and forget about their own desires. This is because you might have had a bad experience when your partner did not seem to enjoy him or herself with you and blamed you. Alternatively, you may feel tired and worried (perhaps about work or children) and focus on helping your partner to have a good time because you don't have the energy to be sexy with them. Therefore, your desire level sinks or soars, while your partner's does the opposite. Concentrating a bit more on what you want can help you to feel turned on and interested in sex. Don't make love focusing everything on your partner rather than what pleases you because they want a certain kind of touch or position. Re-engage with your sexuality by asking for caresses and stimulation you know turns you on. If this seems tricky at first, try the following:

> Ask your partner to play a game. Divide your love-making session into ten-minute sections. Explain that each of you gets a ten-minute segment to ask for whatever they want. Then swap

roles so that the other partner asks. Carry on swapping for as long as you want. Be sure to try out some of the things you might have done in the past, as well as experimenting with new sexual practices that you might have thought about but never experienced.

Pretend you have just met

Put an evening aside to pretend you have only just met. You can start by going out for a drink (but not too many) or a meal, but the object of the evening is to get into bed together. Play the game by imagining you are on a blind date. Ask your partner about themselves and their life. This alone can be an interesting experience as you may find out things you did not know! You should also use the opportunity to flirt outrageously. Touch his or her knee or hand and keep eye contact, occasionally looking down to engage their attention. Wear your sexiest outfit. Women can also use bracelets and earrings to draw attention to their arms and neck. The reason that bracelets are thought to be attractive is that they draw attention to the bare forearm, with its soft and sensitive skin. This is the role of most jewellery – it leads the eye to parts of the body that are erogenous zones in men and women. Once you get back home, pretend you are inviting a new partner in for coffee. Carry on flirting and talking sexily. Say things like, 'I love a man with your sexy eyes' or 'You have a wonderful figure.' Then lead your partner to bed. Undress each other and make love very slowly. Ask what he or she likes and carry out their requests. Afterwards, cuddle up to one another so that you feel close. If some of this game makes you laugh, this is a wonderful bonus. Laughter in sexual relationships is much underrated, but can help you both to feel closer than ever before.

Change the scenery

Explore a change of venue. You have probably heard of the idea of making love in different rooms in your house, other than your bedroom. But a complete change can be a turn-on because it allows you to move out of the roles you have fulfilled at home and be sexier people. Many couples tell me that holiday sex is good because they feel relaxed, but my bet is that it is linked to feeling different about themselves. If you cannot afford a full holiday, consider renting a hotel room for one night (even a local B&B would do). Take a case that is not full of your usual holiday paraphernalia (buckets and spades and baby's nappies). Instead, take several different kinds of lubricants, flavoured condoms (interesting to try out even if you use another kind of contraception), sexy underwear, sex toys, and some silky sheets to put on the bed. Lock the door, put the 'do not disturb' sign on the door and let yourselves go.

You can also try out different venues that have a flavour of the forbidden fruit. For example, did you ever make love or pet intimately in the back of your car? Do you consider that this is behind you now that you are a committed couple? You can rediscover this pleasure by using your garage, if you have one. Ideally, your garage should be connected to the house, but even if it is separate, you can still play out the role of 'teens in the back of the car'. Make sure you are unlikely to be disturbed; shut and lock the garage doors, and get in the car. You can choose whether you leave the garage or car light on or off. Wear your usual outer clothes, but it can be fun to leave your underwear in the drawer. Start by kissing and cuddling, gradually working up to caressing each other under your outer clothes. You may find yourselves giggling at the unusual situation, but this will help you both to feel excited. Push the front seat close to the windscreen so that you have plenty of room for manoeuvre. The woman can sit on the back seat while the man kneels between her legs to enter her (also great for oral sex), or you can masturbate each other to orgasm by hand.

Try pretending

Pretend you are doing something else. This can feel sexually exciting because it has a 'naughty but nice', illicit feeling that good sex often contains. Try sitting next to each other on the sofa (when you can be private and uninterrupted) and put on a video – preferably one with some sexy scenes or with an actor you fancy. Start watching the video, but allow your hand to wander over to your partner's legs and lap. Slide your fingers along their leg, and gradually begin to arouse them by stroking and caressing their penis or clitoral area over their clothes. Keep watching the film, and avoid speaking to one another. Continue the intimate touching until you both feel very aroused. Only then can you turn to one another to continue making love. This game can feel like a test of endurance, but this raises the arousal level because it provides a contrast between the intimate touching and the lack of other contact. You can also try this sitting at a dining table or in bed.

Use music

Make love to music. This sounds simple, but it can be very exciting and quite challenging. You need to pick your music carefully according to the sexual mood you want to create. Soft, relaxing music can help sex to last a longer time; use something with a strong beat to speed up love-making. Try matching the thrust of the penis into the vagina to the beat of the music, or during mutual masturbation match your stroke to the time of the music. You can also aim to get your orgasm to coincide with the climax of the music. If you are into classical music, try matching your orgasm to the highpoint of Elgar's Cello Concerto! Using music in this way during sex is a skill that takes practice, so start with music you know well and about which you feel confident. Rock or rap music can feel exciting and arousing, but match it to your mood so that you both feel up to the demands of this kind of music. Gentler, romantic music usually has a slower beat and can help you both to feel as if you are melting into one another.

Explore painting

Try body painting. Buy some simple children's poster paints (always check at the store that these are non-toxic and safe to use on skin) and a set of differently sized brushes – some with a thick brush for broad strokes, and others thin with a pointed end for detail. Cover your bed in towels with an old sheet on top to protect the linen and decide who will be the painter and who the 'canvas'. If you are to be painted on, remove your clothes and lie on your back or front, according to choice. Now your partner can use you as a canvas. He or she can make separate designs or create a picture. The simplest way to start is to paint long strokes of colour on the limbs and torso. Circle around the nipples and genitals (avoid putting any paint directly on the labia or head of the penis), creating whorls of colour. The human body lends itself to tree shapes, with the body as a trunk and arms as branches and leaves, but any design that you think looks attractive is OK. Your partner will be enjoying the sensation of the brushes running over his or her skin, and your loving attention as you work on his or her body. Once you have finished on the front or back of your partner, you can either paint the other side, or swap over so that you now get the painting treatment. Couples describe this as a very lazy and warm activity, great for a summer's evening when they will be uninterrupted. It is also good to calm you if you have had a period of arguments or unhappiness.

You can make the painting more erotic by praising your partner's body as you paint. Say things like, 'Your breasts are so beautiful' or 'I love the way your bottom looks.'

If you do not want to use the paint because of concerns about allergy, try using different kinds of brushes on the skin, either dry or just with warm water. Buy a range of different bristles, such as baby hairbrushes, men's shaving brushes, and even a new house-painting brush or soft sheepskin paint roller. Never use one you have painted with in the past and beware of anything too stiff or scratchy. Now use the brushes to brush the skin. Try long, up and down strokes on the back, buttocks and legs, alternating with shorter, firmer strokes on the arms and chest. Brush one another's hair (an overlooked pleasure) and continue down over the nape of the neck and shoulders. This kind of brushing is highly erotic and arousing; especially if you then go on to brush the pubic hair. If you are a woman, ask your partner to brush downwards over the vaginal lips (gently, without too much pressure). If you are a man, ask your partner to use a soft brush on the testes and hair around the base of the penis. You can vary this sensation by wrapping a silk scarf around the bristles of the brush. If you want to go on to give a massage, apply the massage oil with a pastry brush. Feathers are also excellent for this kind of sex play. Sweep a long feather (a peacock feather is excellent) the whole length of the body for an electric shock of pleasure.

Discover oral pleasures

Try the pleasures of sucking and licking. I am not talking about oral sex (more on that in the next chapter) but about enjoying the sensuous possibilities of taking fingers and nipples into the mouth. Try dipping fingers in cream or yogurt and inviting your partner to lick it off. If you are doing the licking, take it very slowly, gradually taking more of the finger into the mouth each time you suck the food from his or her finger. Do this with all the fingers, gradually working your way along the hand. You can also drizzle honey or crushed fruit on to the nipples, and then lick off the food in slowly increasing circles. Men are often overlooked for nipple stimulation, but this kind of licking can be very arousing for a man, especially as he watches his partner gently nibbling and licking his chest. You can also kiss mouth to mouth and exchange a raspberry, strawberry or mouthful of alcohol, but avoid putting alcohol anywhere near sensitive tissue as it can sting and cause serious pain!

You can also try toe sucking. Again, dipping a toe in something delicious, and inviting your partner to suck it off can be surprisingly arousing. Always be careful that you have clean hands and feet, with nails trimmed and neat. This is good advice for lovemaking in general as torn nails can tear soft skin and make manual stimulation very uncomfortable.

You can also try kissing and stimulating the highly sensitive areas at the back of the knees or inner elbow. These zones have many responsive nerve endings, but need careful touching if you are to enjoy the sensations. Use the tip of your tongue to lick these areas carefully, describing small circles as you go. You can also use the tip of your finger to stroke these places. Stroke up and down, barely touching the skin so that your partner feels only a gossamer touch. Stroking these areas is not for everyone, as some people say it feels too ticklish, but others say that it creates a sexual buzz that resonates throughout their body. These are also good places to try out brushing or licking.

Case Study catch up

Rhianna and Mark resolved their problems by working on their feelings at times other than in bed. Rhianna learnt to explain to Mark how she was feeling and Mark offered her more affection and tenderness that was not dependent on her returning his approaches with sex. They learnt to resolve the anger they felt outside of sex. They also experimented with different sexual behaviour, allowing them to feel that their sex life was more fulfilling.

Quick tips on sex and anger

● *Always think about where your anger really belongs*. Is it in bed or to do with some other aspect of the relationship?

● *Tell your partner what you enjoy and dislike* in bed rather than hope they will guess or understand without you speaking the words.

● *Never use sex to give your partner a 'message'* about something that has upset you. Sulking or taking revenge through sex is a recipe for a miserable sex life.

● *If you feel your desires never match*, book time out to be together so that sex can happen naturally. Don't push your partner to have sex, but be affectionate and tender so that sex is more likely.

● *Don't be afraid of sexual experimentation*. No one is asking you to do anything you hate, but trying one or two new things could prevent rows of the 'you never want anything different' variety.

- *Stop seeing sex as something you 'give to get'*. Real love-making should be a mutual and shared experience. If you see it as something you trade, or give to keep your partner quiet, you won't get pleasure from sex.

- *Lack of trust or fear about the relationship can lead to anger in bed*. Trace the roots of your uncertainty about the partnership, fix the problem and your sex life will improve dramatically.

- *Relax more and stop stressing about sex*. Sexual anger breeds tension and vice versa. Try only making love on the days you feel relaxed. If you don't have any of these days, do something about it!

- *Tell your partner about any sexual problems caused by past experiences*. This is particularly important if you have suffered sexual abuse or assault. This can cast a long shadow over sexual feelings and it is easy to blame a partner for issues you need to deal with yourself.

- *Express your emotions when they occur*. Saving all your feelings for sex turns it into a pressure cooker of unhappiness and disappointment.

KEY MESSAGE

Anger and sex don't mix. Anger prevents intimacy and creates fear, which can ultimately destroy your relationship.

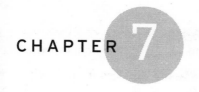

fear and anxiety

. . . .

Occasionally, feeling some fear and anxiety in a sexual relationship is entirely normal. Good long-term sex involves being able to be emotionally intimate with another person, and in order to achieve this we have to be prepared to be vulnerable.

There are always troughs in a relationship when we don't feel confident enough to expose our vulnerable, innermost selves with another person in case we are hurt. As a way of coping, this may mean we shut down on our sexual side for self-protection. Or we may succumb to the temptation of trying to test the relationship and make extra demands on it. We do this in order to check out how prepared our partner is to handle our fears and anxieties.

Learn to sort out your fears

The key to reducing fear and anxiety in any situation is not to make another person jump through hoops; it is to learn how to cope with our own fear and anxiety, rather than expecting someone else to sort it out for us.

Theoretically, sex is a source of joy and mutual support for a couple. It is a way of bringing you together physically, emotionally, mentally and even sometimes spiritually. So what do we have to be afraid of? Why be anxious about something that is so clearly 'A Good Thing'?

The answer is that sex is usually a reflection of our relationship *and* all the other events that are going on for us in our lives. So if we are tired and stressed, if we don't make a deliberate effort to alter our attitude before making love, the sex we'll have will be lacklustre and lethargic. By the same token, if we feel insecure and worried about our bodies, bothered by breasts we feel are no longer youthful and pert, or perturbed by a penis that isn't as firm as it once used to be, we will carry these anxieties into the bedroom with us and sooner or later they will bring us down, draining our confidence and enthusiasm for sex.

The effects of fear and anxiety

At its most basic level, fear or anxiety reduces our ability to concentrate. To enjoy sex, you need to be able to concentrate on pleasure – your own and that of your partner. If you are feeling even slightly anxious, you will find it much harder to experience the pleasurable sensations your body wants to give you. In fact, it is likely that you will be experiencing tension and stress – the opposite of pleasure. And if you begin to have bad sexual experiences because you are worried or afraid, you'll find your sexual appetite plummets quicker than you can say, 'I'm not in the mood.'

Let's look first at the differences between fear and anxiety in the context of a long-term sexual relationship. If you are experiencing real fear because your partner is physically or emotionally abusive towards you, you must ask yourself why you wish to remain in the relationship. Domestic violence can destroy the life of everyone it touches: men, women and children. Living with the fear that your partner may attack you at any moment is no life at all, no matter how much you may feel they love you in other ways.

Violence destroys a rewarding sexual relationship

If violence is the major source of fear in your life, you will never be able to have a rewarding sexual relationship with your partner, simply because a fundamental level of trust between you will be lacking. Some people stay in violent or otherwise abusive relationships for years, sometimes because their confidence is so destroyed by their abusive partner they lose the will to find anything better for themselves.

If you are in a relationship that causes you mental, physical or emotional pain, then you need to analyse very carefully your reasons for sticking with it.

Fear and concern

On a less dramatic note, it is worth pointing out that there is an important difference between fear and anxiety and an appropriate level of concern for the well-being of your sexual relationship.

It is fine to be aware of the ups and downs between you; in fact it is important that you are. But becoming overly anxious or fearful about aspects of your sex life is not so useful, mainly because fear and high levels of anxiety cause your brain to shut down and begin spiralling into unhelpful circles of panic and clouded thinking. As good sex in a long-term relationship is invariably linked to good communication between you, if one or both of you are in a negative spin about something, it will be difficult for discussion and sharing to flow easily between you.

Performance anxiety

One of the major areas of fear and anxiety in sex itself is linked to performance. This is usually a worry that plagues men, but there are women who worry about their sexual performance, too. Nevertheless, most patterns of love-making tend to follow a routine that puts a considerable burden on the shoulders of the man.

This burden is that he should achieve a reliable erection, he must manage not to ejaculate before his partner is sufficiently stimulated to reach orgasm herself, and both parties should time their orgasms so that they climax together. After all, that's what it's like in the movies, so shouldn't we all be matching this ideal in our bedrooms?

The plain answer to this is simple. The above scenario may be what they do in the movies – both pornographic and Hollywood – but Julia and I would say most definitely that it is only *one option* when it comes to what we do in our bedrooms, or wherever else we choose to make love.

And once you realise you have plenty of other choices on offer, what is commonly perceived as the man's responsibility to manage the encounter simply vanishes. This doesn't mean, of course, that he no longer has to bother about pleasing his partner. What it does mean, though, is that you both share responsibility for your sexual experience and for bringing pleasure to your partner. Sex becomes an exchange between loving equals, who don't blame or criticise each other for not 'doing it right'.

Sales of Viagra, the little blue pill that enables a man to achieve a firm erection for several hours, have hit stratospheric heights because they enable men to sustain their erections. While this is a boon for men with medically proven erection difficulties, it does nothing else to improve the quality of a man's love-making. It is crucial that men understand that simply being able to pump away with a firm erection for ages is not the same thing as being a great lover. If you are not careful, your female partner is likely to get bored or sore, or a combination of both, because women are not designed to experience the most intense sexual pleasure solely from receiving a penis in and out of their vaginas.

The clitoris is king, or perhaps we should say queen, when it comes to women achieving orgasms, and men ignore this at their peril. We don't recommend worrying endlessly about sexual performance, but if you want to feel a healthy level of concern about improving your skills as a lover, don't focus on your penis, focus instead on bringing pleasure to your partner in other ways.

Other ways to a woman's sexual pleasure

If this sounds rather unmanly, perhaps I should stress again that a penis is only part of the picture as far as a woman's sexual pleasure is concerned. Try one of the different approaches outlined below, and not only will you be releasing yourself from fear of losing your erection and the unwelcome burden of running the sexual show along very narrow lines, you may well be very pleasantly surprised by your partner's increased levels of enjoyment.

Making love with a 'soft-on'

Yes, it is possible to be inside a woman without an erection, and it is a lot easier than you might think. Some women find the sensation of a man's penis becoming hard after it is inside them extremely arousing. Others simply enjoy the closeness of cuddling up with their partner inside them. This can be difficult to understand for men, who are accustomed to 'doing' in sex. But it really is worth giving it a try if you want to widen your sexual horizons. So, men, follow these suggestions and see what happens:

Make sure your partner is fully lubricated. Ideally use a water-based lubricant inside her and on your penis.

Get on top – gravity helps the blood move into your penis (if you are aiming for an erection) and it is easier to move if you wish. Alternatively, try the 'scissors' position. You replicate the shape of an open pair of scissors with your bodies; the woman lies on the left with the man's right leg between hers, while his left leg lies underneath her.

> Circle your thumb and forefinger around the base of your penis to form a ring and gently squeeze.
>
> Carefully slide your penis inside your partner, keeping your finger ring around the base of your penis.
>
> Squeeze your buttocks to push blood into your genitals if you want an erection to develop.

This 'soft-style' love-making is also rewarding when you are lying side by side in the 'spoons' position, where you both lie on your side with your knees bent, the man tucked behind the woman.

Men tend to forget that they are endowed with several body parts other than their penis that can bring immense delight to a woman. Remember: few women reach orgasm through penetration alone. A man has fingers to stroke his partner's skin and sexual organs, a tongue to lick with, and lips that you can use to caress, nibble and suck.

Skin sensitivity

Research has shown that a woman's skin is ten times more sensitive than a man's, so women appreciate their entire body being taken notice of during sex; not just their genitals and breasts. An inventive lover might use his elbows – great for certain types of massage – or his chest hair rubbed down her back, to make his partner quiver with delight.

Even if you have never experienced an erection problem in your life, which makes you a very rare man indeed, it is worth experimenting with bringing as much pleasure as you can to your partner without using your penis. You will probably be greatly surprised at her enthusiastic response.

(This isn't intended to denigrate the worth of penises, by

the way. They are wonderful. But relying on your penis alone to make you a great lover is a little like judging an entire country on its capital city. Yes, you'll understand the main thrust of the place, but you'll have missed a lot of unexplored countryside that may be equally interesting.)

Sometimes it isn't stress – it's fear

Many people blame their poor sex lives on stress and their hectic lifestyle when they are actually holding back because, at some unacknowledged level, they are in the grip of fear. Below are some of the most common fears that hamper a mutually satisfying sex life with our partners.

A fear of giving up control

Sometimes men withhold intimacy and women withhold sex. The problem with this catch-22 situation is that men don't want to be intimate with a woman who doesn't want sex with them, and women don't want sex with a man who avoids intimacy. This creates the stalemate of a non-existent sex life as a result.

If this is your situation, try instead to think about giving to your partner instead of denying or taking. What may surprise you is that the more you are able to give what they want, whether it is sex or intimacy, the more you will receive what you want.

In her excellent book *The Sex-Starved Marriage*, American couples' therapist Michele Weiner Davis puts it like this: 'In good relationships, people do things for their spouses all the time that may not be exactly what they feel like doing at the moment . . . Real giving is when you give to your partner what your partner wants and needs whether or not you understand it, like it or agree with it.'

This is not about being a doormat or making pointless self-sacrifice. It is about being prepared to make the first step if you want a situation to change. And if your destination is a rekindled and passionate sex life, taking that first step will help enable your partner to join you on your journey together.

A fear of not being 'manly' or 'ladylike'

Rules about the way the sexes are supposed to behave in our society run deep. This is because we have received countless messages, spoken and unspoken, from our families and the world around us, about the way we are supposed to behave sexually. Men are not supposed to be emotionally vulnerable, for example, and yet for many men, having a sexual relationship with someone else opens up their vulnerabilities.

Acknowledging your fears and the depth of your love for a woman is not thought by society to be a masculine virtue. You only have to look at the so-called 'lads' magazines' to get the message that women are fine for sex, but a bloke's most intense relationship is with his football team or his car. While this attitude may bring comfort to men who find it hard to establish successful relationships with women, it does them no favours in the long term.

Often men find it a welcome relief to play a less actively masculine 'doing' role in their sexual relationship, and couples can have fun swapping over the 'dominant' and 'submissive' roles between them. Equally, women can be frightened of exploring their assertive side when it comes to sexuality, and some can feel that looking as if they enjoy sex will make them seem wanton or even sluttish. Firstly, some men adore wantonness and sluttishness, and, secondly, a good sexual relationship allows you to experiment with all sides of yourself, without fearing that you will be judged and condemned by your partner.

If, somewhere in the back of your mind, you feel 'nice girls don't like sex', ask yourself where that belief comes from. The likelihood is that it originates from a parent or teacher, and to be fair to them, it is probably something that they were told to believe, too. But *you* don't have to believe it, especially if you find that it is limiting the pleasure you experience in your sexual relationship.

Try replacing it with the belief that 'nice girls have great sex', and take steps to make sure that it is true. Research shows that the quickest way to change how you feel about something is to take action. Rather than sit around and wait to feel differently, take a small positive step to embrace your new belief and it will soon start to feel real for you.

A fear of losing control

This is often linked to fear of challenging the limiting gender roles described above, and a worry that if you act outside them your partner will be appalled and flee from the bedroom. So it might mean that a man feels a wave of emotion rush over him, but is frightened to express it. Or a woman might be anxious that an orgasm that makes her shake, sigh or scream will terrify her partner. (Some women also worry that their make-up will get smudged and their hair will get messy.)

The truth is that the majority of women are delighted when a man who is making love to them experiences a rush of emotion, and every man in the world yearns for his partner to have an orgasm that makes her shake, sigh and, ideally, scream with ecstasy. (That way he knows she's having a good time and, handily, it confirms his prowess as a great lover to the neighbours.)

By the same token, a woman who is reluctant to kiss in case she spoils her lipstick, or who hesitates to give oral sex in case he notices her roots need attention, is misunderstanding the basic nature of most men. An ideal sexual mate for a man doesn't need perfect make-up, a perfect figure or perfect hair colour. All she needs is to be enthusiastic about having sex with him. And believe it or not, seeing a woman with wild hair and streaked make-up after having sex is a much underestimated source of male pride.

A fear of being overwhelmed

If your childhood relationships weren't entirely helpful, and particularly if you experienced a troubled relationship with someone who looked after you when you were young, there is a chance that entering a sexual relationship as an adult may make you feel fearful that somehow you will be sucked into a relationship that will destroy your sense of self.

People who experience this unpleasant sensation build barriers in order to protect themselves; but as good sex is about openness and connection, a person who is emotionally defensive is unlikely to experience real passion. If you feel you or your partner has psychological blocks which are hampering your mental and physical connection, it may be wise to seek counselling as a couple, which can be an effective way of challenging and rooting out damaging experiences from your past.

A fear of remembering pain from the past

You need not have experienced anything as potentially harmful as sexual abuse to find sex awakens memories of embarrassment or humiliation that you would rather forget. Trying to bury these memories won't be possible at the same time as trying to build a satisfying and rewarding love life with your partner. Some people find that therapy helps them come to terms with experiences they would not have chosen for themselves. Others manage to 're-frame' past incidents and choose to feel differently about them.

I was greatly heartened to hear the story of the reaction of one woman who had been raped in her own home by a hooded attacker. When he escaped through a window, she dressed and went to a friend's nearby flat to call the police. The policeman was astounded by her composure, which didn't leave her throughout the coming weeks and months. Someone asked her how she managed to handle her dreadful experience so well. She replied: 'Do you think that I'm going to allow ten minutes with that bastard to wreck my whole life?' Exceptional maybe, but it shows it can be done.

Also, this isn't about burying feelings and denial – this woman now works with and supports other women who have been raped. It is making a choice about the view you take of the events in your life. We can't control what happens to us, either as children or even as adults. What we can choose, though, is our reaction to it. If you have had a bad sexual experience in your past, you don't have to allow it to blacken your sex life for ever. Talking to a trained psychosexual therapist or counsellor can help a great deal. And making the choice to feel differently about it can be an empowering experience too.

A fear of loss and rejection

When you allow someone else inside your heart, you open yourself up to the prospect of pain. For some people this is just too frightening to contemplate. As a result they lead lives that are free from passion and commitment.

As you'll probably have gathered after reading the earlier chapters of this book, your sex life is not something that is separate from the rest of your existence. If you are emotionally distant from your partner, if you lead a life that is routine, and you rarely plunge into excitement and adventure, the chances are that your sex life will be a reflection of this.

If you are looking for a more passionate love life, you have to be prepared to care deeply about your partner. And if you are very close, that also means that you may have to face the much more painful prospect of losing them one day. Shutting down on your feelings to immunise yourself from hurt is not a satisfactory way to deal with this.

If you can appreciate that your partner brings you joy, but that you are whole and complete in yourself, the possibility of losing them is no longer petrifying, it is simply sad. And you will cope. You can make the choice to be the sort of person who is OK with themselves, and therefore able to love someone else without being frozen by the fear of losing them. Or you can allow the terror of rejection and the possibility of loss to paralyse you in the face of passion.

The fear of giving an inch . . .

. . . and being taken for a mile. Some women worry that if they begin to be more sexual with their partners, they will end up having to be sexual all the time. This is particularly common in relationships when one partner has a higher libido and desire for sex than the other. The low-desire partner fears that if they appear to increase their interest in sex, it will be the first step on a pathway to continual sexual demands that will make them feel cornered and exhausted.

For some men, it can be the fear that being more intimate and expressing the emotional side of passion will lead to the requirement that they will have to talk all the time and will have no private space or time to themselves any more.

What individuals coming from both perspectives need to know is that neither fear is likely to be fulfilled. It is only when one partner is withholding either sex or intimacy on some level that it seems to them that the appetite of their other half is insatiable. What many couples don't understand is that when you refuse to satisfy a partner's basic needs and desires, it creates an exaggerated sense of neediness in the other partner.

If a man is reluctant to talk, and a woman pursues him, constantly stressing her need for communication, she may well find that he retreats even further. But if she allows him a little space when he first gets home, for example, and asks when it would be a good time to talk, the chances are she will get a much more positive reaction.

The same policy of non-pushness applies to sex, too. A man or woman who feels sexually frustrated by their partner's lack of desire may try to turn every affectionate touch into something sexual, so keen are they to increase the amount of time they spend sexually with their partner. What they don't realise is that this behaviour simply drives lower libido partners in the opposite direction, and conveys the message that sex is wanted all the time.

In reality, once the partner's needs have been satisfied sufficiently, the demands will diminish and a more comfortable balance between you can be established. But you both need to be able to put your fears to one side and trust that this will happen.

A fear of becoming a sex god or goddess

Strange as this may sound, there are people who shut down on their sexuality because they fear that once unleashed it will be uncontrollable and they will find themselves attracted to people other than their partner. Sex is a powerful force inside us, but it is not uncontrollable. People who fall 'in lust' are making a choice, even if they pretend to themselves that they are simply carried away by the force of their emotions.

Yes, once you become involved in a passionate relationship with your partner, you may find that you are more attractive to other people. This is because people who radiate sexual energy are noticed by others. But you don't have to act on this. You can make a mature decision how to act. In fact, if you are already in a passionate, committed relationship with your partner you are much less likely to be tempted away by someone else. As the movie star Paul Newman once said of his wife, Joanne Woodward, 'Why go out for a burger when you have fillet steak at home?'

Overcoming fear and anxiety

Fear, anxiety and worry eat away at a relationship. They produce muscle tension, pain and problems with concentration. Of all the issues that can affect a successful sex life, anxiety is the one that can have an almost immediate effect. If you return home after hearing that your job is in jeopardy because the firm you work for has financial problems, only to hear that your partner has been told that his or her elderly mother is seriously ill, sex is likely to be the last thing on your mind. Moreover, if worry is chronic, lasting for months rather than hours or days, sex can gradually slip down your list of priorities so you do not make love at all. This can lead to a feeling of distance and coldness between you, causing sex to be less likely or very mechanical when you do get together.

CASE STUDY ·

Gina and Barry

Gina and Barry have been married for eight years. Gina is a self-employed translator of university textbooks whereas Barry is a house-husband, caring for their two small daughters. Their financial situation has always been variable as Gina can earn a lot or little depending on the jobs she takes on. They find that when money is tight they both worry about the implications. Will they be able to pay the mortgage? Can they afford new shoes for the children?

Gina has noticed that this affects their sex life. She finds it very hard to relax and enjoy sex when she feels this way, and Barry seems to withdraw emotionally when they go through their periodic anxieties about cash. Gina also admits that she has always been a worrier, and that her mother was, too. In the early days of their marriage, Gina worried that she was 'no good at sex' and that

Barry thought she was boring, although Barry has reassured her that this is not the case. But when her working life is under pressure, her old fears return. Barry also struggles with his anxieties about Gina getting pregnant again, because their second daughter was not planned and they found it very hard to manage for months after her birth. This means he sometimes cannot get an erection when he wants to because he unconsciously fears impregnating Gina.

Consequently, their sex life is often tense and unsatisfying. Barry and Gina would like to feel more relaxed and less fearful about sex, but are not sure where to start.

First steps

If, as you read this scenario, you recognise any elements of your own worries about sex here are some ways to overcome the anxiety and fear that affects your sex life:

- **Avoid 'globalising' your situation.** By this, I mean that anxiety is worsened by seeing it as all-consuming. Often, anxiety spreads gloom over everything that seems important. For example, Gina and Barry feel that their unreliable cash situation infects everything they do. If this happens to you, try to 'shrink' the worry to what it really changes in your relationship. Allowing a concern to spread over a wide area can only happen because you allow it to.

- **Be practical.** Unfocused worry often leads to a feeling of impotence (it's no mistake that we use impotence to mean lack of erection as well as a lack of control). For example, if you have money worries, sit down with your accounts and bills and work out what needs to be done to tackle the concern. Agree who will do what and ensure you carry out your decisions. Don't be afraid to get help from others who can advise you.

● ***Break the anxiety down into smaller, bitesize, issues***. If you find it overwhelming to cope with a large worry, make a list of all the elements of the concerns that are causing you trouble. Now put it into the order that you need to do things. You probably know you do this for mundane things, such as DIY, but it can work for emotional troubles as well. For example, if you know you need to talk to your teenage daughter about her drinking with her mates, make a list of the things you want to say, and what order you will say them in. You may want to talk to your partner, decide if she should be told she cannot see her friends for a while, and so on. Adopting this strategy helps you feel less occupied by the concern and opens up the possibility to enjoy sex in a more relaxed way.

Anxiety linked to sex

But what if your anxiety is actually linked to sex itself? For example, two very common concerns are body image and sexual performance. You may also fear being close, physically and emotionally, to another person. This can often result in unsatisfying casual sexual encounters or an avoidance of sex altogether.

Try the following to relieve these kinds of fears and anxieties: ask yourself 'What am I afraid of?' You may fear commitment, giving control to a partner or letting go of your own control in bed. Alternatively, you may fear that if you allow your partner to know you as vulnerable (sexually needy, for example) they will somehow take advantage of you.

Try this exercise:

> Write a list of the issues that cause you trouble in bed, with a note on why the item can cause difficulties. For example, here is a typical list:
>
> - Having sex in any position other than face to face. *My partner gets annoyed because he or she wants more variety.*
>
> - Turning down a request for sex. *My partner is hurt when I say 'no'.*
>
> - Leaving the light on. *I feel uncomfortable about my body shape/size.*
>
> - Saying 'I love you' or being affectionate towards my partner. *I think he or she may see me as weak.*
>
> - I need to be in control. *I worry that if my partner takes more control I might have to do things I won't like.*
>
> Once you have your list, look carefully at the 'reasons' you have given for the things you do. As you read them, formulate a challenge in your head. Imagine you are someone else who has to come up with a reason why these reasons are faulty. To steal some words from the Dr Pepper advert, ask yourself 'What's the worst that could happen . . . if I try to be more relaxed about the items on the list?' For example, take the item about leaving the light on. Your challenge might be 'My partner has never said my body turns him or her off. In fact, he or she often says I am sexy' or 'Perhaps I am anxious about my body because I am not confident about other areas of my life such as socialising or working effectively.'
>
> Go through the whole list in this way. Once you have challenged yourself, decide on one action for each issue. For

example, you might decide to try leaving the light on next time you make love, buy some aromatic candles to soften the light in the room where you make love, take up swimming to tone your body so you feel better about yourself or talk to your partner about your feelings. As you gain in confidence, look for more ways of varying the items you feel scared about and add practical changes. Do this slowly, trying out one change for a while before moving on to another challenge. Gradually, your fears and anxieties will reduce.

It is possible that you will uncover some issues that are not so easily solved. If, for example, you realise that you often find it difficult to reach orgasm because you do not truly trust your partner, you will need to think through what you want to do about this situation. You can still use this 'action' method, but it might involve seeing a relationship counsellor or therapist (www.relate.org.uk and www.basrt.org.uk has lists of Relate centres and therapists near you) to help make up your mind about taking appropriate choices.

Your guide to oral sex

If Val and I had taken a poll among our clients over the last few years on what caused the most anxiety during love-making, oral sex would come close to the top. Many couples seem to encounter difficulties with this aspect of love-making. Some people just don't want to do it, whereas others feel that their skill is poor or that they have never figured out exactly what you are supposed to do. This could be due to the idea that oral sex is something recently invented by modern culture because of the coverage it gets in magazines. Women's monthlies and men's magazines often carry features on 'how to give a good blow job' or how to 'lick your way to success with a woman'. This seems to have given many couples a feeling of inadequacy over giving or receiving oral sex. In fact, oral sex has been part of love-making since ancient history and is a perfectly natural thing to do. Before the media started telling us that there was a good or a bad way to give oral sex, people just got on with it!

The other problem with oral sex is that couples worry about the 'unclean' element. This is because, in men, the opening of the urethra at the tip of the penis is also the opening for semen to pass through, and, in women, because the openings to the urethra and anus are relatively close to the vaginal opening. Some men and women find the idea of licking or kissing around this area uncomfortable, fearing that they may inadvertently discover urine or faeces in, or close to, the vagina, or penis. So before we go on to discuss oral sex, let's clear up this cleanliness issue. If you bathe or wash well before sex, you will not find either urine or faeces in the genital area. Men should pull down the penile foreskin to make sure that the area around the glans (the tip of the penis) is clean, and should wash their bottom and anus. Women should wash the vaginal area, taking care to rinse the labia well. They should also wash the anus and whole bottom area. If you find soap irritates you, use warm water and a sponge, use a bidet, or take a shower. Direct the showerhead over the penis or into the vagina to ensure the whole area has been thoroughly rinsed. This will ensure cleanliness and allow you to kiss or lick the genitals with no problems.

However, you should bear in mind that oral sex with someone you don't know well, or whose sexual history is unknown to you, can run the risk of causing a sexually transmitted infection. This is because infections can enter through small cuts in the mouth, infecting the person giving the oral sex. Herpes (the cold sore virus) can be caught from genital herpes; AIDS can also be caught through oral sex. If you want to give oral sex to a male partner you are unsure of, always use a condom. You can also purchase a latex barrier film to place over the labia and clitoris so you can give oral sex, while protecting yourself from catching a disease. The golden rule is: if you are at all unsure of your partner, don't give or receive oral sex. Nevertheless, if you feel secure with your partner, don't let issues about cleanliness put you off what can be a highly arousing experience.

Oral sex is a highly arousing technique in love-making. It is also a very intimate act, perhaps more so than intercourse. If you use the steps below you will gain in confidence, making fellatio and cunnilingus a natural and exciting part of love-making:

How to give a man oral sex (fellatio)

Ask your partner to sit or lie on his side, on the bed. Some men also like to stand so that the woman sits on the edge of the bed or chair during oral sex, but if you want your confidence to grow, this position can feel a little intimidating. You can start with a flaccid penis (some women like to take the whole soft penis in their mouth to feel it become erect), but if you want to give oral sex while using a condom, your partner will need to be erect first.

Hold the base of the penis firmly but not too tightly, and bring your lips down to the tip of the penis. Using your tongue as if you were licking an ice cream, gradually lick around the tip of the penis. Pull the foreskin back (if he has not been circumcised) and concentrate on licking the area around the frenulum – the small piece of skin that joins the foreskin to the head of the penis (this may be missing if he has been circumcised). This area is extremely sensitive to touch and most men find it highly erotic to have it caressed. You can vary the shape of your tongue by relaxing it so that it is soft and gentle, or point it, making the tip harder, to give little dabs of touch around the head of the penis.

When you feel confident, open your mouth a little to form a soft 'O' shape and take the head of the penis into your mouth. Be careful not to catch the penis on your teeth. It can help to push the penis head slightly to one side so that it rests against your cheek.

In this position, you can suck and move the penis around in the mouth and against the tongue. Be gentle, unless your partner asks for firmer licking or sucking. Rocking your head slightly can help the sensations to simulate thrusting in the vagina. You can do this quite vigorously, taking more of the length of the penis in your mouth. Notice that I am not suggesting you immediately try to take the whole of the penis into your mouth. Many women worry about this because they fear they will gag if the penis hits the back of the mouth. Most men enjoy the sensation of being sensuously licked and sucked rather than a full-on thrusting into the mouth, although you may want to try this when you feel more comfortable about oral sex. Ask your partner to lie still rather than trying to push his penis into your mouth, and to relax while you stimulate him.

The next question that usually arises about oral sex (if your partner is not wearing a condom) is 'What if he comes in my mouth?' This is really a matter of personal choice. There is nothing in sperm to harm a woman, even if you swallow it (it has about the same number of calories as a serving of broccoli!) but the sensation is not to everybody's preference. The taste of your partner's sperm will vary according to what he has been eating. Curries and rich food will give it a strong flavour; a simpler diet will render it almost tasteless. But it is not the taste or texture of sperm that usually causes the problem. It is the anxiety about a bodily secretion present in the mouth. We have natural defences against taking anything that exits the body into our mouth. There are good biological reasons for why we feel disgust about this. Avoiding others' secretions protects against catching diseases or infections, and this taboo has been present for millennia. This is often the true reason for women avoiding taking sperm into the mouth, and explains why no matter how often books like this one, or their partner, tells them that it is OK, women still avoid doing it. The important thing is, whether you choose to allow him to come in your mouth is *your* choice. Never let a man tell you that this is what every woman does or blackmail you by telling you that you are no good at oral sex if you won't do this. In fact, if he behaves this way, why are you having sex with him in the first place? If you don't mind your man ejaculating into your mouth, try moving the penis away from the back of the mouth when he lets you know he is about to come. This way you will not get a shot of ejaculate at the back of your throat, causing you to gag. If you don't want him to come in your mouth, ask him to tell you when he is close to orgasm, and lean your head backwards while continuing to rub his penis with your hand. Some men like to see their ejaculate on a woman's breasts, so you could move your body to achieve this at the moment of ejaculation.

Once you feel more confident about the basics of oral sex, you can add some variety by using some simple props. The most common is to coat the penis in something good to eat – honey, cream, chocolate spread or crushed soft fruit are among the most popular. Icing sugar or cocoa powder, lightly dusted over the penis and testes is fun, and sometimes called the 'cappuccino effect'. Flavoured condoms are good if you need to use a condom. Look for fruit flavours and different colours to add interest.

You can also try different positions:

Ask your partner to sit on a chair with his legs apart so that you can kneel on the floor to perform oral sex. In this position, he can also thrust gently into your mouth. Remember to soften your mouth to avoid collisions with your teeth. You can vary how much of his penis you take into your mouth by moving your head forwards or backwards, matching his thrusting. If you feel the need to control the speed of thrusting, hold the base of the penis. If he lies on his side on the bed, you can encourage his thrusting by putting your hand on his bottom, pushing it into your lips and mouth. These techniques help you to maintain some control while also giving your partner the experience he wants. If your mouth gets tired from being open, just pull your head away for a few minutes while maintaining hand stimulation.

When giving oral sex it is not always easy to keep your own level of arousal alive. You can improve this by using a vibrator. As you stimulate your partner, place a vibrator between your legs, or rub your clitoris with your free hand. In this position, a vibrator will give you a pleasantly low level of clitoral arousal, increasing your pleasure while you please your partner.

You can also lick and kiss the testes, but be careful not to pinch the soft skin in this area, as it can be very painful for your partner. Some women find they can take a whole testicle into their mouth, but gentle licking and sucking around the testes is usually just as arousing for your partner.

How to give a woman oral sex (cunnilingus)

Ask your partner to lie on the bed with a pillow tucked under her bottom so that her pelvis is tilted upwards towards you. She should lie with her legs slightly apart, but not stretched out so far that the labia are pulled apart. This is because many women enjoy the erotic sensation of the labia brushing against each other during love-making. As the labia swell during stimulation (a natural response to arousal), she may wish to part her legs a little. Some women like to pull their legs up so that their feet are placed flat on the bed level with their knees; others prefer their legs to lie straight out.

First, use your fingers to stimulate the clitoris gently. Stroke up and down the inner and outer lips while blowing gently on the whole area. Use soft breaths, allowing the air to play over the vaginal area. This is a delicious feeling – both subtle and playful.

Using the tip of your tongue, gently lick along the vaginal lips. Vary the strength of your licking by changing your tongue from soft to hard. Gradually approach the clitoral area, using your tongue to circle the clitoris. It can help if you use your finger to brush the labia aside from the clitoris, but some women find this too intense a sensation, so be guided by her response. Use soft kisses and licking as you cover the labia and clitoris. Imagine you are licking the juice from a melon or mango, relaxing your lips and mouth. You can also nuzzle the area at the top of the thigh where it meets the labia. Brushing your hair (or the top of your head if you are bald) along this zone adds to the stimulating sensations.

Once you have got used to using your tongue in this way, try flicking your tongue over the top of the clitoris. This is the 'butterfly' technique and has a teasingly arousing effect on the clitoris. Ask your partner to hold her labia apart so you can concentrate on this area.

Some men also want to know if they should put their tongue in the vagina. There is nothing wrong with doing this, and it can be arousing. Ask your partner if she would like to try it.

At first, just insert the tip of your tongue, working up to pushing your tongue in further. You can also use a finger placed in the vagina to aid this technique.

As with male oral sex, once you are confident about the basic technique you can add other things to increase the fun. Try smearing some honey, cream, yogurt, fruit juice or a flavoured lubricant on the labia. Take your time licking it off and reapply if you are both enjoying it. You can alter position by the woman standing with her legs apart while the man kneels beneath her, or she can crouch over his face while he licks her from a lying down position. The woman can also try having all her pubic hair removed to improve the sensation of oral sex, but this is a potentially painful procedure that she should feel happy about undertaking. Many beauty salons provide this service (often called a 'Brazilian').

As with women who find the idea of bodily secretions unacceptable, some men also worry that they will find the natural lubrication a woman produces during sex unacceptable. These secretions have no flavour, except some saltiness, and a musky scent. This scent contains a pheromone that acts as a turn-on during sex, so, far from being distasteful, the scent should be an aphrodisiac.

If the woman has any problems with coloured or smelly secretions, she should not have oral sex and should see her GP. Do not give a woman oral sex if you have any doubt about her sexual history. It is probably best to avoid oral sex during the woman's period, although some couples do find it acceptable. This is an activity you need to feel confident about after gaining experience of giving cunnilingus at other times of the month. Never be pressurised into giving a woman oral sex if you know it is not appropriate. If she demands it, and you are unhappy about it, you need to work on your whole sexual relationship rather than give in to her demands.

Many men enjoy bringing their partner to orgasm through oral sex. It is likely that she will move around and could grip your head with her thighs. Hold her legs and lift your head up a little to give your nose clearance so that you can breathe properly if this happens to you.

Past experiences

Another source of anxiety and fear is the effect of past experiences on the relationship you are in at the moment. If you had a difficult childhood, perhaps even suffered sexual abuse (and as many as one in five people report having an inappropriate sexual experience as a child), you may find it affects your sexual response. You may be psychologically poised to defend yourself, and this can make fulfilling sex very difficult, even when you know you care deeply for the person you want to make love to. Following the advice on relaxation earlier in the book may help you, but expert therapy can greatly help with sexual trauma. Always ensure that the therapist/counsellor you choose is a member of a reputable counselling organisation (the British Association for Counselling and Psychotherapy, the British Association of Sexual and Relationship Therapists are well known and set strict criteria for their members) and that the counsellor has experience in dealing with sexual trauma.

Case Study catch up

Gina and Barry found they were able to enjoy sex more by working out what they needed to do to about contraception. They decided that Barry should have a vasectomy to prevent his worries about getting Gina pregnant again, that Gina should look for a part-time job that gave them some continuity of cash flow and that they would buy a 'sex guide' video to help them explore new ways of being sexual together.

Instant anxiety fixers

- ● *Practise relaxing more by taking time out for yourself.* Do something you need to concentrate on as this can prevent anxious thoughts.

- ● *Undertake some light exercise.* Walking, swimming and cycling are all good for your physical and mental health. Exercise releases endorphins (a natural relaxant) that can prevent anxiety. The government recommends 30 minutes a day five times a week to improve fitness and well-being.

- ● *Break a problem into 'bitesize' pieces.* Tackle each part until you have resolved the issue.

- **Challenge your thinking about sex**. If you regard it as a competition, or a way of getting what you want, you are denying yourself the love-making you could have.

- **Take action**. Worrying about how you will feel if you leave the light on during love-making, or feeling guilty because your partner has asked you to leave it on and you have refused, is much worse than experimenting with a low light or candle. OK, you could hate it but you will never know unless you try it out.

- **Lack of trust in a partner is a desire killer** and is bound to make you anxious. Think about why you do not trust him or her and then decide what you want to do about this. For example, you may decide to talk to him or her about your feelings, examine what has led to the lack of trust, or assess whether the relationship can continue. (Read Chapter 8, Trust and Security, for more help on trust.)

- **Believe in yourself as a sexual person**. One of the chief sources of anxiety about sexual relationships is a lack of confidence in being sexy. Think of it this way. My experience as a sex therapist for over 18 years has told me that most people derive only half the pleasure they could from love-making. Those that have a satisfying sex life are not the most beautiful, or with the best figure or even the most intelligent. They are those people who believe themselves to be capable of responding in a total way to love-making with their partner. This is often a private pleasure that perhaps even close friends may not suspect, although this 'essence of sexuality' often shines through.

- **Your fear and anxiety is limiting you**. Every day you allow yourself to worry is like wearing a ball and chain. Challenge the basis of your fears and the chains will fall away, allowing you to live a life free of chronic anxiety.

KEY MESSAGE

Fear and anxiety can eat away at a successful sex life. Challenging the basis of your worry and taking appropriate action can give you the love life you have always wanted.

CHAPTER 8

trust and security

· ·

Trust and security are necessary bedfellows; it is hard to have one without the other. But they are not the same thing. In most couple relationships, trust comes from a sense of security. Trust is the essential building block for a relationship to flourish and grow.

Sustaining physical passion

The key to sustaining physical passion is not to let trust dwindle into complacency. Trusting your partner because you can't imagine anyone else being attracted to them, for example, probably means that you've stopped seeing them as a vibrant, sexual being yourself.

The difficulty with maintaining trust in a relationship is that we rarely have a conversation with our partner about what trust means to us. Most of us assume that in a good relationship we should be able to trust our partner not to hurt us physically or emotionally, to behave in a responsible, adult way and not to enter into intimate, physical relationships with other people.

But these rules may not apply to everyone. In some European cultures, for example, husbands and wives may have discreet affairs, but they trust that neither of them will do anything to break up the family unit. Understanding what trust means to you is an important part of establishing your relationship, and it is worth reassessing on a regular basis.

Expectations from family life

When a couple gets together, both bring unspoken expectations from their families and their early lives, and these 'family rules' or traditions play a much greater role in their union than they would like to think. Mutual expectations of trust are often unspoken, but still rank highly in our checklists for an important relationship.

If you think you've cast off the shackles of your family, and your relationship began with a clean slate, there is a one-word answer that will probably prove that, sadly, you are mistaken: Christmas. How you celebrate or don't celebrate Christmas, whether you are a Christian or not, will have had a profound impact on you and will have an impact on relationships you have in the future.

Rules about when to open presents, what to buy as presents, who gets presents, all collide when a couple first get together and try to satisfy themselves and two sets of families with different expectations. Which is why thousands of people are to be found not in front of log fires or round the glittering tree on Christmas Day, but tearing up and down motorways, trying not to get indigestion from eating two family Christmas dinners.

The effects of our upbringing

Psychologists make much of 'attachment theory', which boils down to the idea that much of our adult behaviour is governed by how successfully we were parented as babies and young children. If our needs were met regularly, we will probably have grown up feeling reasonably secure and able to trust other people. If, on the other hand, we were ignored or even neglected as infants, as adults we will find it hard to trust others.

This is, of course, only a theory, and there are many stories of people who have lived lives of real deprivation who have nevertheless managed to grow into wise and loving adults who have made good relationships with others. So whereas it isn't helpful to think it is inevitable that it will be hard for a neglected child to trust as an adult, it may be useful for you to explore this issue if you feel that you have difficulties in this area. You can do this either on your own or with a therapist you like and find rewarding to work with.

Do you want to rekindle your sex life?

If you are trying to rekindle a sex life with your partner, you may find it useful to ask yourself three questions before you start:

1. Do I respect this person as a good friend?

2. Is my life better with this person than without them?

3. Do I want to grow with my partner and do I trust them to be there for me?

If the answer to any of the above is 'no', the chances of experiencing passionate sex with them once more – or even for the first time – are low. This is because passion in a long-term relationship is not dependent on the cocktail of chemicals released in your body when you first fall 'in love', but depends on the quality of your relationship *outside* the bedroom.

The bad news is that you have to sort this out first, and it can be hard work. The good news, though, is that when you do put time and effort into your relationship so that your partner becomes a good friend who supports you as an individual, the benefits of your improved relationship are very likely to include a much richer and more rewarding sex life. (It then becomes an upward spiral: better sex means a better relationship; a better relationship means better sex.)

The Magic Five Hours

If you feel at a loss and don't know where to begin, you could do worse than take on board the advice of the US marriage guru John Gottman, author of *The Seven Principles for Making Marriage Work*. He points out that to improve the quality of your relationship significantly, you need to spend just five hours concentrating on each other during the course of a week. He calls it the Magic Five Hours and this is how it works:

- *Goodbyes*: before you say goodbye to your partner in the morning, make sure you've learnt about one thing that is happening in their life that day – whether it is a doctor's appointment or lunch with a former colleague. (Allow 2 minutes a day x 5 working days: 10 minutes.)

- *Hellos*: make sure you share a stress-reducing conversation at the end of each work day. Take it in turns to listen to each other without offering advice and suggestions, unless asked. (That's 20 minutes a day x 5 days: 1 hour 40 minutes.)

- *Offer unsolicited admiration and appreciation*: this isn't as shallow and artificial as it might sound. We all need positive verbal and physical strokes to keep us going. It need only account for a few minutes a day. (Say 5 minutes a day x 7 days: 35 minutes.)

- *Give affection to each other*: how long is it since you caught your partner by the waist and kissed them like you meant it? Always try to kiss before you go to sleep, and let go of any stress between you at the end of the day. Long night-time conversations are not a good idea as they are likely to stop you sleeping soundly, but if something is niggling you, resolve to put some time aside to talk about it the next day and be generous with your goodnight kiss. (Say 5 minutes a day x 7 days: 35 minutes.)

- *Make a weekly date*: just two hours a week on your own, having fun rather than discussing domestic details, will reinvigorate your relationship far more than you might think. Book a babysitter if you have children, and choose one night a week where you do something as a couple that you both enjoy. Don't try to split up the time into single hours, or even half-hours scattered across the week. You need a solid block of time in order to relax properly with each other, and make sure you decide what to do beforehand, otherwise you'll waste valuable minutes debating how to spend your time.

The grand total of the above is just *five hours*. John Gottman believes that working briefly on your marriage every day will do more for your health and longevity than working out at a health club. Whether you believe this or not, it will certainly help your relationship to flourish and you will feel more emotionally connected to each other. From there it is only a few short steps to reconnecting physically.

An exercise in intimate trust

Once you have established a trusting relationship with your partner, try this exercise when you next make love. It is very simple to do and is about making an intimate connection:

At the point of orgasm, look deeply into your partner's eyes. Most of us close our eyes and retreat into a world of our own sensations when we reach orgasm. Sharing your orgasm with your partner is a loving and trusting thing to do. There is no need to repeat this every time you make love, but give it a try at least once and observe the effect it has on you both.

Affairs can happen at any stage

No discussion of trust in relationships can be complete without a mention of affairs that can happen at any stage of a couple's life together. People tend to think that affairs are all about sex, and one partner succumbing to temptation, while the other remains an innocent victim. The picture is much more complex than this.

Couples who arrive for counselling after an affair often say they'd like to 'turn the clock back', and for everything to be as it once was. But if they did this, the chances are an affair would happen again. *This is because an affair is a symptom that something is not right in the marriage; it is not the cause.*

Most marriages continue after an affair

According to the couples' counselling agency Relate, two-thirds of marriages continue after the revelation of an affair. The successful ones usually accept that there were hidden problems in the relationship before one or other of them began an affair. It takes enormous courage for both partners to admit this, especially for the so-called innocent party, as friends and family tend to see affairs as a black and white issue, with the person who has had the affair being universally condemned for behaving badly.

Certainly, having an affair is not a good way to highlight that there is a problem in your relationship; there are dozens of better ways of handling it. But for some people, it is an unconscious response to a situation that is not satisfactory, and if the couple are to stay together, it is essential that *both* individuals are prepared to analyse what wasn't working in the lead-up to the affair.

The fallout

Even if the couple do eventually decide to stay together, the initial fallout from the revelation of an affair can be devastating.

For most of us, our trust in our couple relationship involves being sexually faithful, and to discover that this trust has been betrayed can feel overwhelming at first.

Perhaps surprisingly, sex can suddenly become very passionate, as it may be invested with the fear of losing someone you love, or even from a desire to outperform another lover who has threatened the relationship. Alternatively, the betrayed spouse may feel like shutting down on sex altogether, and often sex is the last thing to return when a couple choose to stay together after an affair.

How to handle the discovery of an affair

There are five steps you can take that can help you handle the fallout from an affair:

1. Don't sit up all night talking about it. Fix short times to discuss it, rather than allowing your conversations to go on for hours on end. You will both end up exhausted. Instead, try to decide what you have gained from each of your discussions. It may help you to make a note of any issues you have discussed and made a decision about.

2. Limit discussion about the affair to half an hour a day. Be prepared to use an alarm clock or the timer on a mobile phone, if necessary. During this time, one partner can ask questions or both can talk about their feelings. Be prepared to listen to the other without interruptions or accusations. At the end of half an hour, stop the discussion. This requires considerable discipline, but it will help you both cope better in the long run.

3. Only ask questions you can handle hearing the answers to. When you first find out about an affair, you may be tempted to ask thousands of questions, ranging from 'Why?' to 'Is the new lover better in bed than me?' Pace yourself, and ask yourself first how helpful it will be for you to hear the answer to the question you want to ask. If you are the person who has had the affair and your partner asks you why it happened, take the trouble to think through your response. Don't just reply, 'I don't know, it just happened.' Offer whatever you think may have had some impact on your decision to have the affair in the first place: something like 'I felt lonely after the baby was born' or 'I was worried about losing my job.'

4. Don't blame the lover. It might seem handy to label the lover 'man-mad' or a 'seducer' and to focus your anger on him or her. But if you do shift responsibility for the affair on to the lover, you are denying yourself the opportunity to explore why the cracks in your own relationship occurred. And you are increasing the chances that an affair will eventually happen again.

5. Give yourself time. Don't make any response like 'pack your bags and leave' for at least three days. You need time to assimilate the news, and making immediate decisions is not a good idea. Try to have a couple of good nights' sleep before you issue any ultimatums. Neither should you expect to sort out the repercussions from an affair in a few weeks. You may both long for the wretched business to be over, but you have to bear in mind that recovering from an affair can take months or even years. Feelings of grief, jealousy and anger may surface at unexpected moments in the future, and it's a fair bet that some of these uncomfortable

feelings will arise when you make love together. Rather than being embarrassed and caught off balance by this, accept that these feelings are natural and part of the healing process in terms of your couple relationship. Acknowledge them and then let them go.

When a secure relationship seems dull

For some people, being in a secure sexual relationship sounds deadly dull. These are people who thrive on the thrill of the chase, the uncertainty that accompanies the first flush of romance and the rush of powerful bonding hormones that unite you in the early days together. As a relationship settles, these people become restless, wonder to themselves 'Is this all there is?' and head off in the direction of a new lover who can offer the highs and excitement of a new relationship. These individuals who love 'falling in love' bounce from one relationship to the next usually because they fear building a sense of commitment and trust with someone else.

Underwriting this attitude is a fear of loss. They have a horror of becoming too close to someone and having to come to terms with all this entails. They would rather be in love with an ideal man or woman for a short while and move on, than grow an enduring love for a real person with all the flaws and minor disappointments they will inevitably bring. For such people, the word 'security' sounds more like a prison cell than a safe haven.

People who are happy only when everything is unpredictable not only may fear making a commitment to you but they are also deliberately sabotaging your attempts to get to know them. They set up a smokescreen of uncertainty, which prevents the relationship ever reaching a mature level. Some people choose to hang on in this kind of relationship, forever hoping that, one day, life will settle down. But it rarely does.

If you are in a relationship with a person who fears making any kind of commitment, ask yourself, 'What am I getting from this relationship?' Is your partner's refusal to commit to you actually giving *you* the chance of maintaining some distance in a relationship? How would you feel if they turned around tomorrow and said they really wanted to settle down with you for ever? Or do you feel deep down that you don't deserve a 'proper' relationship and that you are lucky to get what's on offer, no matter how unsatisfying it may be for you?

If you find that the one thing your partners have all had in common is an inability to enjoy a trusting and secure relationship with you, it is likely that there's something inside you that needs to change. Unreliable partners may be reflecting an unconscious belief you hold about yourself. Think back to your childhood. What were your relationships like with your parents, for example? Did either of them act in a way that you found hard to trust? If you've been let down as a child, your adult self may be choosing people who will let you down, because that's what you've learnt happens in relationships. Try to think this through; you may want to talk to a close friend about it or sort it out with personal counselling.

Extreme predictability kills passion

On the other hand, extreme predictability is stultifying and the antithesis of what a passionate relationship is about. Always making the same moves physically before you make love, for example, is a guaranteed way to extinguish your partner's desire for you sooner or later. But you do need to show some predictability in your relationship, so you are free to explore on your own and in your relationship, rather than being eaten up with uncertainty and confusion.

Qualities to look for in a sexual partner

If you want a trusting sexual relationship, look for these qualities in your partner:

- *A relatively even temper*: this doesn't mean that they can only manage one note, emotionally speaking, and they should be able to express strong feelings when it is appropriate, but they shouldn't veer wildly from one extreme emotional state to another.

- *Being capable of following some routine*: we are not talking Horlicks and a biscuit at bedtime every night here, but if your partner says they feel smothered by any kind of routine, they are probably indicating that the relationship is not for them. Someone who turns up when they say they will, and can follow a schedule, if necessary, generates a feeling of trust.

- *Matches deeds with words*: sounds obvious, doesn't it? But plenty of people make empty promises; they may even mean what they say at the time, but the reality turns out to be hollow. Don't expect a great sex life with someone who lets you down on a regular basis. The trust, which enables you to be adventurous and explore new things together, simply won't exist.

Jealousy

The opposite of security is insecurity, which is a fertile breeding ground for jealousy, one of the most destructive emotions in a relationship. Excessive sexual jealousy can wreak havoc in a relationship, scarring both partners, and often paving the way to the end of the relationship, which is usually what the jealous person most fears.

Nine times out of ten, jealousy is born of insecurity and low self-esteem on the part of one half of the couple. If an affair has been revealed, it can seriously damage the self-esteem of the partner who has been betrayed and they may react by questioning their judgement in all things, not just their relationship.

Jealousy grows when one partner invests everything in their other half, and comes to depend on them for all their good feelings. The threat of losing them, therefore, seems terrifying, as the loss of their partner would mean the loss of their whole existence.

The only way to exorcise jealousy is to work especially hard at building up your own life, so that you learn to gain happiness and fulfilment from sources other than your partner. This might mean taking up a hobby you find rewarding, or taking time to invest in friendships that you might have let slide when you first met your partner.

If you are a jealous person, try to understand that the key to holding on to someone you love is to make yourself the kind of confident, attractive person they would choose to be with. Neediness and a tendency to try to control someone else are not appealing characteristics. Keeping your relationship secure is not about fencing in your partner with rules and restrictions, but doing everything in your power to keep your relationship a safe space to which you can both retreat whenever you wish.

Jealous people often find it hard to relax and 'let go' in a relationship. If you are prone to jealousy, mull over these definitions of 'letting go'. You may find one or two are especially helpful:

Letting go

To let go is not to cut myself off; it's the realisation that I can't control another.

To let go is not to try to change or blame another; it's to make the most of myself.

To let go is not to care for, but to care about.

To let go is not to judge, but to allow another to be a human being.

To let go is not to be in the middle arranging all the outcomes, but to allow others to affect their own destinies.

To let go is not to be protective; it's to permit another to face reality.

To let go is not to adjust everything to my own desires, but to take each day as it comes and cherish myself in it.

To let go is not to deny, but to accept.

To let go is not to criticise and regulate anybody, but to try to become what I dream I can be.

To let go is to fear less, and love more.

Building trust in sexual relationships

Sex without trust is nearly impossible. The most rewarding and satisfying sex you can have is when the love-making you enjoy allows you to feel emotionally attached and able to trust your partner. Imagine the difficulties of trying to make love if you were always wondering what your partner might do next or if they cared for you at all. Of course, it is possible to delude yourself into thinking a sexual partner *is* trustworthy, usually because you want it to be true. In this situation, time and events will inevitably prove if your desires have a solid basis or are just a hopeful dream.

CASE STUDY ·

Paul and Kelly

Paul and Kelly are both 28 and have been together for two years. They have always had an 'up and down' relationship and have split up twice. But something has always brought them back together. Kelly finds it hard to examine why this happens. She feels strongly about Paul. He is witty and entertaining, but can be unreliable and difficult to deal with. Their sex life is variable, sometimes passionate, at other times cool or non-existent. Paul knows he wants to be close to Kelly, but also fears being tied in a long-term commitment. They go through a dance of intimacy, sometimes close to one another and sometimes distant. Kelly is also not completely sure if she wants to be with Paul in the future, but is drawn to him.

Kelly knows that Paul has affairs. He has never made a secret of his flings and none of them have lasted more than a week or so. He often tells her they 'are just sex' and Kelly feels she has no right to ask Paul to be faithful when neither of them knows what they really want. But this does affect Kelly during love-making. She often has trouble achieving orgasm and can find it hard to relax. Sometimes she fakes orgasm to avoid discussing the issue with Paul. Paul also feels uncomfortable about sex, wondering how Kelly really feels about him, and can find it difficult to feel turned on.

. . . .

Paul and Kelly have never examined their relationship or their sexual responses, other than to say something like 'This is just how we are.' This leaves them struggling to trust one another. Their relationship skates the surface, never allowing them to feel fully involved with the other. The consequence is that they spend time together feeling vaguely unsatisfied and unfulfilled. Sex can feel a bit mechanical because neither of them is willing to give themselves in a complete way, so that the sensations are often thrill-seeking rather than rewarding at an emotional level.

The link between sex and trust

Although you might get a momentary thrill from sex where you feel unsafe, in a long-term relationship trust equals good sex. Trust means not only knowing your partner is not going to run off with your best friend, or run the credit card up to the hilt, but also that you can let him or her caress you in a way that arouses you. In order for this to happen, you need to literally let him or her into the secret places of your body. You need the confidence to say what you want and to know that these needs will be met, at least some of the time. You also need to know that if you say you don't want to do something that this will be respected. Sexual security is a two-way street. Your partner needs to know that if they do this for you, then you will do the same for them. Trusting sex connects to respect – if your partner respects your body and your feelings about sex they will not push or force you into anything you would hate, and vice versa. This does not rule out experimentation in sex. This can be a good thing, but you should remember it is only an experiment, which by its nature needs to be tested. If either of you hate what you have tried out, then trust will flourish if the other accepts this conclusion rather than sulking if the experiment does not continue.

Developing sexual trust

There are several aspects that you can work on to develop sexual trust:

Know yourself

If you understand how you feel about sex and its role in your life, your ability to trust a partner will increase. For example, if you rely on your partner to give you the ideal sexual experience, rather than understanding your own sexual response, you are bound to be disappointed and mistrustful next time you make love. Explore your own body, learn about how your body works during sex, and ask for what you like.

Know your partner

When you first make love with a new partner, feelings of excitement and novelty will probably give you good sexual experiences. This feeling can last for a few weeks or months. However, eventually you will need to explore what pleases your partner and what sex means to them. For example, do they like to make love frequently or infrequently? What sort of touching do they like? And, where do they like to make love (bed, lounge, back of the car!)? You may learn a lot of this along the way, but asking him or her what they want and how they feel can help you to gain a sense of trust in your partner.

Respect one another

All sexual trust is based on respect. If you respect your partner and they respect you, sex will feel safe. I am not suggesting that this means it has to be boringly predictable with only one position and only on a Saturday night! Safe sex is not only about wearing a condom (although this is an important part of safe sex practice), but more about feeling you can relax, feel aroused and reach a climax without fearing your partner might do something you would find uncomfortable or distinctly unarousing. This means you need to tell one another what you feel happy about and what you feel is unacceptable. For example, you may be completely happy with oral sex but your partner may feel unsure.

If you push and demand that they share your pleasure you are not respecting their feelings. Not to mention that your nagging will probably prevent them from even considering oral sex. You might consider gently introducing him or her to the idea by suggesting you try it in the shower (many people who refuse oral sex do so because they fear that they, or their partner, may be 'dirty' because the vagina and penis are close to the urine outlet) or just for a brief time to assess how it feels. Some people try to bully their partner into following a sexual practice they want by saying, 'Everybody else does it. You are the only one that is refusing.' This will not gain you your partner's respect or encourage them to do what you want because they will either feel a loss of self-esteem, preventing them from doing what you ask, or dig in their heels in order to counter your bullying. Neither of these are a basis for a healthy sex life between equal partners. If you know that you sometimes bully, or receive sexual bullying of this kind, ask yourself or your partner if you are making the mistake of regarding sex as a series of exercises that end in a climax rather than an expression of love for one another. Try not having penetrative sex for a couple of weeks. Instead, have sexual evenings when you caress and stroke one another, talk about love-making and watch some sexy films together (but not porn as this can prevent the kind of intimacy you are seeking). This kind of 'sex break' can give you the time and space to reassess what you want really from love-making.

Restoring sexual trust

If you have been through a breach of trust, it can feel very difficult to resume a sexual relationship. Not only will you feel that without trust sex is difficult but you will also feel reluctant to make love to someone you fear could hurt you again. You could avoid sex, literally push your partner away, or question whether you ever want to sleep with them again. However, men and women can have other responses to lack of trust. If your partner has had an affair, you may find yourself making love in order to prove that you are as good as his or her lover. You may also feel dissociated from love-making – as if you are watching yourself having sex, but not fully involved. This is often especially true if you are trying to put a marriage back together and believe that sex is a duty – one of the things you 'should do' to improve the situation.

So how can you resume sex after a breach of trust?

- *Take things slowly*. Snap decisions not to have sex, or to pretend nothing has changed, are usually born out of shock, and fear that you cannot sort out the situation. If you have recently discovered an affair or your partner has deceived you in some other way, but you want to stay together, you need time to get used to how you feel about sex.

- *Go back to the beginning*. It is no good assuming that you can pick up your sex life where you left it. The sexual relationship you had in the past is over and cannot be the same. Now is the time to re-imagine what you want from your love life. It can help to book dates together, as you might have done when you first met. Build up to love-making after several weeks or months of re-establishing your relationship. Over a period of time, start with kissing and cuddling, moving to intimate touching and, finally, intercourse.

- *Don't be afraid of your feelings*. It is common for couples who have been involved in an affair to try to crush their feelings when it comes to making love again. If you are to regain your trust, you need to acknowledge these feelings rather than deny them. It might help to write feelings down or talk to your partner (but not during sex if you can help it). If you find you 'freeze' during love-making because images of your partner's ex-lover come into your mind (a not unusual response) just breathe slowly and imagine the picture dissolving. If this happens frequently, you are probably attempting to resume sex too fast after the affair and need to slow down. But it can still happen years after the event. It is important to tell yourself that it is you he or she has chosen to be with and concentrate on the physical sensations rather than the thoughts about what happened months or years ago.

- *Ask 'open questions' about sex*. This point in your life is like a blank page. If you are starting again then you now have space to talk about your love life. If anything positive can be said to come from an affair, this is it. A good way to start is to ask 'open questions' about sex. An open question is one that requires more of an answer than just 'yes' or 'no'. For example, you might say 'Tell me what time of day you prefer to make love?' instead of 'You like making love in the morning best don't you?' Alternatively, start your questions with why, how, when, where and what. These all allow your partner to answer questions in a more open way. Here are some starter questions to help you open up the subject of sex with your partner:

Where do you most like me to stroke you?

What's your best time of day for love-making?

How do you want me to hold you?

When do you feel closest to me?

What gives you most pleasure during love-making?

You will gradually come up with your own questions. Don't deliver them as an interrogation. Be loving towards one another and ask the questions carefully and gently. Allow your partner time to answer. You can even play a game, taking turns to ask each other a question. While you are in this period of redevelopment, you can also consider exactly what you want from sex. For example, you may want to think about, and challenge, who usually initiates sex, the time you spend on love-making and what you actually do during love play.

This kind of talking and action allows trust to develop. As you put together a plan for your sexual life together, you will be testing out whether your partner is reliable, can offer warmth and empathy and if what they hope for from sex is also what you want. If there is disparity, try not to worry. Talk about the areas where there are difficulties and look for compromises that allow you both to feel you have something of what you want.

Danger signs

Trust can take a long time to develop in a sexual relationship after it has been broken. If you encounter the following in any sexual relationship, you may need to think hard about whether you want the relationship to continue:

- Your partner refuses to talk about changing any element of your sex life, wanting everything to be exactly as it was, even if he or she knows you are unhappy about this.

- They keep elements of their life hidden from you and you wonder if they are still seeing someone else.

- Sex feels much worse than before. Alternatively, sex feels very hyped up and strange. Either of these effects may indicate your partner is finding it hard to commit to you.

- Sex feels as if it is separate from the rest of your relationship. For example, you may argue frequently and feel worried about the relationship, but still have sex. Don't kid yourself that if you are having sex the relationship is OK. It is probably under great pressure and the sex is still hanging on as the last intimacy you have left.

- Your love life feels routine or is missing altogether. Your partner, or you, make excuses to avoid love-making.

If you identify with these statements, you need to talk about what is happening in the relationship, as sex may be acting as an emotional barometer, telling you there are serious problems. Find a therapist or counsellor near you (www.basrt.org.uk or www.relate.org.uk) for help in unravelling your problems.

Your guide to starting again

If you have had a long break in sexual activity, perhaps as the result of an affair or some other betrayal of trust, starting again can be difficult. Alternatively, you may be restarting your love life with a new partner, seeking to learn to trust him or her and regain your own sexual feelings. Many people ask therapists, 'When is the right time to begin sexual relationships after a break?' There is no hard-and-fast rule that says you should resume sex after six weeks or six months. Your decision will depend totally on your feelings and the state of the relationship – this is especially true after an affair. Some couples panic and try to have sex straight away. Often this is because of the anxiety of the person who did not have the affair trying to compete with the assumed attractions of the lover. On the other hand, the person who had the affair may initiate sex in order to appease the partner and recompense for the situation. Panic sex is not a good idea. Neither of you will have worked out what you want from the relationship. Trying to indulge in intercourse – the most intimate thing you can do together – will only confuse things further. In addition, as time goes by, you may regret rushing things and wish you could have slowed down the whole process.

Other couples pursue the absolute opposite of this approach. They stop touching one another and avoid any physical contact. While this is perfectly understandable after an affair, the coldness you build up, especially if you want to try to stay together, can freeze your emotions and sexuality so that neither of you has a clue how to become close again.

Here are some ideas on redeveloping physical closeness if you want to rebuild your sexual relationship:

Timing

Consider the timing of being sexual together. For example, Louis and Diana wanted to restart their sexual relationship after a temporary separation. Louis had not had an affair, but they had been very unhappy, with plenty of arguments. They had agreed to have three months apart, meeting up again after this time. When they met, Louis was tempted to sweep Diana into bed, but Diana resisted his sexual overtures. She told him that she needed to get to know him again and to feel she could trust his commitment. Instead, they agreed a series of 'dates' where they were not physically intimate but spent time talking about the relationship and their sex life.

The best way to judge whether you feel you want to resume sex again is to ask yourself how you might feel *afterwards*. If you detect any possible feelings of regret or ambivalence, you should wait a little longer. This judgement can be muddied by the memory of what has passed between you before, so try to think about the relationship as a new start. Imagine you have just met your partner, and use all the faculties you would normally employ in meeting someone for the first time. If you want a rough rule of thumb on time, give it at least three months after a break up or affair before thinking about sex. In reality, it will take longer than this to assimilate your experiences, but if you tell yourself it will be this long you are less likely to dive into bed together because you want to prove yourself or pacify your own guilt.

Starting again

Once you have decided that you are ready to start again, how should you go about it? The best way is to think yourself back to the early days of your relationship. Even if you began your sexual relationship very quickly after meeting, there will have been a period of flirtation and touching before you had intercourse for the first time. Think of this process as a ladder that you can step off any time you wish.

On the first rung of the love ladder is seduction. Usually we think of seduction as one person seducing the other, but in real life, most seduction is mutual. It might not always look this way to the outsider, but it usually involves a 'come on' signal from one partner, with a 'come here' from the other partner. You need to give your partner the right signals so that they know you are serious about sexual matters. How you do this is very personal, but you could consider a sensuous candlelit meal together, a picnic on a warm day or an evening stroll to look at the stars.

Touch them frequently on the knee, shoulder and hands. If you think things are going well, stroke their face, and kiss them on the forehead or neck. *Then stop!* The temptation is to carry on so that soon you are in bed again. But you are on a journey, and this kind of seductive event is designed to be part of the testing process. It can help to sleep apart from your partner during this time so that you have a clear thinking zone as you consider how you feel about being intimate again. You may need to make this clear to your partner as they may see the first rung as a sign that things are 'back to normal'. As advised earlier in the chapter, during this time continue to talk and assess why things went wrong in the past.

Early experimenting

The second rung of the ladder is to recreate some teenage behaviour. Most teenagers experiment with touching and caressing before going on to have intercourse at a later date, either with the same person or with another partner. Often this kind of touching is done with clothes on for fear of discovery. Now you need to build up to petting with your partner.

Choose a time when you can be alone, and begin by kissing and cuddling. You may prefer to do this away from the bedroom. Kiss your partner tenderly and gently at first, caressing their body through their clothes. Run your hands over their body, concentrating on the hips and chest. Unbutton and undo shirt collars, blouses or trouser zips. Try to keep as many clothes on as you can – just pretend you could be disturbed at any time. Explore beneath his or her underwear and arouse them by rubbing the clitoral area or penis while they are still dressed. It may take several sessions to get to this stage of intimacy, but once again *stop*. This may seem a false halt sign. You could think, 'If we can do this why don't we just have full sex?' The reason you need to stop now is to keep the feeling of exploration and newness. If you leap into bed, this feeling will be lost and your new start jeopardised.

Resuming intercourse

Now you can begin to think about moving to having intercourse again. Once more, find time when you can be relaxed and uninterrupted. Make sure your room is ready (see Beat your stress demons in Chapter 4, Stress, for ideas on getting your room ready for love-making), and lie down together. You may prefer to be semi-clothed, or in some attractive nightwear, but now is the crucial moment for you to reconnect. Your love-making this time must be carefully handled. Don't slip into the patterns you followed before (with this partner or any other). Be tender and loving towards one another.

It can help to start love-making with a massage. Use scented oil (baby oil is OK but avoid contact with the genitals as it can cause dryness and discomfort) and massage each other all over the body. Concentrate on the shoulders, back and neck, as this is where tension is often held. As you caress each other, tell your partner how you feel about him or her. Let them know you want to be emotionally close to them as well as physically close. Say something like, 'It's wonderful to be with you again like this' or 'I want our love-making to reflect how we feel about each other.' This is important because without it you might both wonder exactly what the sex means – does it mean we are back together or is this just an interlude before we finally make up our minds? Of course, you might decide even after sex that the relationship cannot continue, especially if things between you deteriorate. For now, though, try to connect deeply with your partner. Let yourself trust that the relationship has a future and that sex will be a warm and satisfying experience.

After your massage, spend a lot of time caressing one another. Avoid trying novel sexual positions or techniques that you think might impress each other. Instead, stick to positions where your bodies are fully touching most of the time. Kiss one another and stroke one another's face and hair. Kissing eyelids, earlobes and the nape of the neck is very touching and says, 'You are special and important to me.'

As you move towards intercourse, use the missionary position or one where you are in full body contact with one another. This will help to cement your closeness to one another and tells your partner that you are not looking only for 'sensation-based' sex but for 'relational-based' sex – in other words you want to make love to them, not just have a sexual experience that you could have with anyone.

Use a lubricant to ease the penis into the vagina. This is because after any gap in love-making you may need some extra help to resume intercourse. The vagina does not shrink in any way, but if you are older than 30 it can lose its elasticity slightly between acts of intercourse, particularly if the sexual abstinence is more than six months. You can remedy this by inserting a finger while bathing or using a penile-shaped vibrator while you are not having sex, but any minor difficulties are normally overcome once you resume regular love-making. Remember to use a condom if you have stopped taking the pill or any other form of contraception during the break. If your partner has had an affair that was sexually intimate, you should consider using a condom because it is not possible to know whether their lover carried a sexually transmitted infection. This probably sounds a bit tough, but we have met several women whose partner infected them with an STI after an affair. If either of you have any doubts, see your GP for tests or referral to a specialist clinic, which can offer counselling and advice on this issue.

The final step

The last rung of the ladder is what you do after making love:

> When you have finished, spend time cuddling one another. Stroke each other and ensure body contact. Tell your partner

how special they are and how important it was to you to wait until sex could be this good. If you wish, you can describe the love-making as a fresh start, the beginning of your new life together or use any words to mark the occasion as different from all the other times you have had sex together. You could also bring a drink to bed or some special food after love-making to celebrate your togetherness.

As you go on to develop your newfound sexual relationship, you will gradually gain in confidence and want to experiment with some old favourites – sexual positions, for example – or try out new things that you might have read about in this book. While you are in this introductory phase, talk to one another about your love life, explaining what you like and dislike. While you are rebuilding in this way it is important to emphasise that you need to work on the intimacy of sex, not just the goals of orgasm and ejaculation. In fact, if you have been goal-orientated in the past, it could be this attitude that is spoiling your sex life. See sex as part of your whole relationship, reflecting your growing closeness, rather than something you 'bolt on' to your everyday partnership.

Resuming sex after a break can be difficult. If you take the staged approach we have outlined above you should find it is much smoother and less traumatic than worrying about how you will behave if your partner asks you to go to bed. Avoid the 'nought to 60 in ten seconds' approach. Instead, climb steadily to the sexual speed you feel comfortable with and you will reap the benefits as you pause at every step. This approach will also give you space to decide if you want to go on to the next rung of the ladder. If you find that the relationship is not what you wanted or decide to slow things down a bit, you will have the benefit of knowing that you can do this without regret.

Case Study catch up

Kelly and Paul found that thinking about whether they knew them-selves and each other was a real revelation. They discovered that they actively avoided understanding what sex meant to each of them. Paul told Kelly that he felt sex was no different from a meal with someone, whereas for Kelly it had an investment that was far more emotional. Reluctantly, they decided to split, as they realised that they had different goals in sex and in relationships in general.

Quick ways to sexual trust

- *Always be alert to the context of your relationship*. For exam-ple, if you want a close relationship and your partner seems to want something different, convincing yourself he or she may change their mind and see things from your point of view could set you up for a disappointment.

- *Always practise safe sex*. Use a condom and know your part-ner before jumping into bed. Protect yourself by telling friends or relatives where you are going and with whom, especially if you intend to stay overnight.

- *Take time to establish sexual relationships*, either in a new partnership or in one where you want to start again after a dif-ficulty. Trust takes time to build up, and giving yourself time to learn about your partner can prevent nasty surprises later.

- *Maintain a good sense of sexual self-esteem*. If you feel you are not worth much, or not much good in bed, it won't be a surprise if your partner treats you the same way. You deserve to trust your partner. If you feel you can't, but think you should put up with their behaviour, you will never have the loving sex you crave.

- **Stroking and caressing your partner**, telling him or her what you like and varying your sexual routine help to build trust. This is because you are offering to be vulnerable by saying what pleases you. They should return this compliment. This shared sense of loving vulnerability creates a feeling of trust as time goes by.

KEY MESSAGE

Trust needs working on throughout the whole of a relationship. Sexual trust is about letting go of your usual barriers and defences, allowing another person into the most intimate parts of your body and mind. If you can achieve this, even after a breach of trust, you will create a satisfying relationship.

afterglow

. . . .

Having great sex should send you off to sleep – or out to work – with a warm heart and a smile on your face. Hopefully, reading about *How to Have Great Sex for the Rest of Your Life* will give you a similar boost. The message of this book is that it is possible to have a rich and rewarding sex life, irrespective of the number of years that have passed since you first met . . . or the number of wrinkles on your face or the amount of cellulite on your thighs.

You will also have had the chance to reflect not just on the quality of your sex life but also on the other vital ingredients of love, trust and understanding that make up the whole of your relationship.

If your sex life has ground to a halt in recent weeks, months or even years, hold on to the fact that it does not mean it is finished for ever. As the previous pages have revealed, with a small amount of effort and determination it is possible to rekindle desire with a long-term partner and to go on to experience what may be an entirely new dimension of passionate, committed and exciting sex.

The key to reinvigorating a tired sex life is not to expect too much at first. If you've given up hope of your husband, who offers only a swift peck on the cheek, ever sweeping into the bedroom and announcing he is crazy with desire for you, it may take a reasonable amount of time before you can build his (and your) sexual confidence. And if you are tempted to get carried away wishing that your partner would behave differently, never forget the role that you play in the relationship.

Remember that if you are a woman who wants her partner to be a more exciting lover, you have to ask yourself, 'What is my contribution towards exciting sex with my partner?' If the answer is, 'Well, it's just something I think about' then it is time to consider the suggestions in this book for improved communication, because no man can mind-read what you want sexually (or in any other aspect of your relationship, for that matter).

Equally, if you are a man whose wife truly believes that her varicose veins and grey hair deny her the right to feel good about herself in bed (and out of it), you will need plenty of love and patience to convince her that it is her that you truly want, and not just the act of sex itself. But it can be done. Boosting your partner's self-esteem with genuine, heartfelt compliments is one of the greatest gifts you can give a woman, which comes with the added advantage that it doesn't create a debt on your credit card.

Sex is the same as any other area of life, in that although a goal might seem distant it does not mean that it is not worth achieving. So don't shrug your shoulders and accept that a fading sexual relationship inevitably comes with the territory in a long-term partnership. It does not. Take small steps, and concentrate on what works for you both; discard what doesn't. Of course, you are unlikely to move from the sexual equivalent of Sunday league football to the Premiership overnight. But if you concentrate on making small changes one at a time, and allow the effects of these to filter through before you add to them, your progress should be steady and sure.

The best way to make and maintain any kind of change is to communicate your thoughts and feelings about it with your partner. Build a vocabulary that allows you to talk about sex. It may feel clumsy or awkward at first, but persevere, and you will soon begin to reap the rewards of being honest and open with each other.

When we see couples that are struggling in their relationships and with their sex lives, there is usually one common thread that they share. And that is they have either lost – or never acquired – the knack of being emotionally intimate with each other. Being emotionally intimate with someone means sharing your thoughts, feelings and fears at a deep level, safe in the knowledge that your partner will love and accept you for who you truly are.

If you have stopped doing this (or perhaps you have never done it), it means that your conversations are restricted to things outside your couple relationship, rather than inside it. You may be preoccupied with work, your home or your children, but you probably pay very little attention to what is going on between you as a couple.

If you rarely share your emotional reactions, or restrict yourselves to expressing only negative or blaming thoughts, invisible barriers will grow between you. And the chances are that sooner or later sex will end up lacking in meaning or passion for both of you.

Use the tips and techniques in this book by themselves to perk up a flagging sex life, by all means – you may have found that some of the suggestions have worked already. But if you take time to create emotional intimacy between you as well, you will ensure that the improvements in your sex life are built on a firm foundation of mutual respect and love.

One final word here for the benefit of holding on to a sense of fun. Couples receiving therapy to improve their sex lives often report back anxiously that they did a certain exercise and it made them giggle, and they ask, 'Is this OK?' The answer is that it is more than OK – it is absolutely fine. Of course, laughter can be a cover for embarrassment, and it helps if you can both acknowledge this. But it also plays a valuable role in bringing you closer together. Laughter is a positive reminder that great sex is about love, pleasure and joy – and sex can be a source of all three blessings throughout the whole of your life.

further reading

Julia Cole, *Crunch Points for Couples*, Sheldon Press, 1997

Julia Cole, *After the Affair*, Vermilion, 1999

Julia Cole, *Make Love Work for You – an essential guide for career couples*, Hodder & Stoughton, 2000

Julia Cole, *Loving Yourself, Loving Another*, Vermilion, 2001

Julia Cole, *Find the Love of Your Life*, Hodder & Stoughton, 2001

Julia Cole, *How to Stay Together Forever*, Vermilion, 2003

Dr David Delvin, *Love Play*, Ebury Press, 1994

Melanie Fennell, *Overcoming Low Self-esteem*, Robinson Publishing Ltd, 1999

Suzi Godson, *The Sex Book*, Cassell Illustrated, 2002

John Gottman, *Why Marriages Succeed or Fail*, Bloomsbury Publishing Ltd, 1997

John Gottman and Nan Silver, *The Seven Principles for Making Marriage Work*, Orion, 1999

Mark Greener, *The Which? Guide to Managing Stress*, Which? Books, 1996

Cathi Hanauer (editor), *The Bitch in the House*, Viking, 2002

Sarah Litvinoff, *Better Relationships*, Vermilion, 1991

Sarah Litvinoff, *The Relate Guide to Sex in Loving Relationships*, Vermilion 2001 (first published 1992)

Joseph LoPiccolo and Julia Heiman, *Becoming Orgasmic*, Piatkus, 1999

Dr Patricia Love and Jo Robinson, *Hot Monogamy*, Piatkus, 1994

Barry and Emily McCarthy, *Rekindling Desire*, Brunner-Routledge, 2003

Lyle H. Miller and Alma Dell Smith, *Stress and Marriage*, Pocket Books, 1996

Anne Nicholls, *Make Love Work For You*, Piatkus, 2002

Dagmar O'Connor, *How to Make Love to the Same Person for the Rest of Your Life and Still . . .*, Virgin Books Ltd, 1985

Val Sampson, *Tantra: the Art of Mind-blowing Sex*, Vermilion, 2002

Rachel Swift, *Women's Pleasure*, Pan Books Ltd, 1993

Rachel Swift, *Fabulous Figures*, Pan Books Ltd, 1995

Michele Weiner Davis, *The Sex-Starved Marriage*, Simon & Schuster, 2003

useful addresses

British Association for Counselling and Psychotherapy
BACP House
35-37 Albert Street
Rugby
Warwickshire CV21 2SG
General enquiries, tel: 0870 443 5252
Email: bacp@bacp.co.uk
Website: www.bacp.co.uk

British Association of Sexual and Relationship Therapists
PO Box 13686
London SW20 9ZH
Tel/fax: 0208 543 2707
Email: info@basrt.org.uk
Website: www.basrt.org.uk

Institute of Psychosexual Medicine (IPM)
12 Chandos Street
Cavendish Square
London W1G 9DR
Tel: 0207 580 0631
Email: ipm@telinco.co.uk

Relate
Herbert Gray College
Little Church Street
Rugby
Warwickshire CV21 3AP
Relate Central Offices (general enquiries), tel: 0845 456 1310
Relate Line, tel: 0845 130 4010
Relate Direct, tel: 0845 130 4016
Website: www.relate.org.uk

index